# Private Practice for the Mental Health Clinician

**Stanley Kissel**

Rochester Mental Health Center



AN ASPEN PUBLICATION ®
Aspen Systems Corporation
Rockville, Maryland
London
1983

Library of Congress Cataloging in Publication Data

The author has endeavored to provide drug administration guidelines that are in agreement with current literature. It is suggested that appropriate information sources be consulted when dealing with new and unfamiliar drugs. It remains the responsibility of every practitioner to evaluate the appropriateness of a particular opinion in the context of the actual clinical situation with due consideration to any new developments in the field of drug administration.

Kissel, Stanley.
Private practice for the mental health clinician.
Bibliography: p. 301.
Includes index.
1. Psychotherapy—Practice. 2. Mental health services—Marketing. I. Title. [DNLM: 1. Community mental health services—Organization and administration. 2. Private practice. 3. Psychology, Clinical. WM 21 K61m]

RC455.2.P73K57 1983 616.089'0068 82-24445
ISBN: 0-89443-8492

Publisher: John Marozsan
Editorial Director: R. Curtis Whitesel
Executive Managing Editor: Margot Raphael
Editorial Services: Eileen Higgins
Printing and Manufacturing: Debbie Collins



Library of Congress Catalog Card Number: 82-24445
ISBN: 0-89443-8492

*Printed in the United States of America*

1 2 3 4 5

*To a loving family*
My wife, Pearl
My three children, Steven, Neal, and Elizabeth
From a fortunate husband and father

# Table of Contents

# Preface

During the past fifteen years a wide variety of mental health practitioners have expressed interest in independent practice. Academicians such as sociologists, social psychologists, learning theorists, and anthropologists have begun to leave their "ivory towers" and provide professional service to the public. The rising costs of goods and services have given impetus to salaried professionals to pursue part-time independent practice with greater interest. Finally, there has been an eager clientele looking with great expectation to mental health practitioners for help in solving some of the many dilemmas, such as family conflicts, stress, and delinquency, that have plagued our society during the second half of the twentieth century.

Recent writings addressed to the practitioner have placed great emphasis on the business aspects of private practice. Professional skills and competency have been relegated to a minor position. *Private Practice for the Mental Health Clinician* aims to remedy this situation by taking a transactional point of view regarding business person-professional polarization. We will avoid the pitfalls of business versus professional skills and competency and instead describe the practical and productive impacts wise business practices have on professional conduct. We will delineate how skillful and competent clinical procedures can help establish and maintain successful independent practice. We will examine the challenges—headaches and all—posed by independent practice, and suggest some possible and effective strategies available for meeting them, whether making the leap from student to independent practitioner or going the route of full-time agency worker to part-time private practitioner.

The first chapter suggests a number of key personal and professional issues that clinicians considering independent practice are wise to come to terms with early in their professional careers. The next two chapters are devoted to the multitude of business considerations facing the independent practitioner. They consider in detail ways of meeting these tasks.

Chapters 4, 5, 6, and 7 describe the multifaceted ways part-time and full-time clinicians can structure their practice to maximize new referral sources, keep old referral sources, and enhance diagnostic and intervention technique. Chapter 7, on how to go about giving community talks, should be most welcome by the clinician inexperienced with this marketing approach. Sample talks along with step-by-step instructions for the construction of a community talk are included.

In the belief that individual and community education is an essential responsibility of the mental health practitioner, Chapter 8 contains annotated references of books and films for adults, children, and parents. Chapter 9 presents a discussion of drug therapy. Such a chapter was included because of the increasing number of patients being medicated and the concomitant need for mental health practitioners to be knowledgeable and resourceful in collaboration with their medical colleagues. Of course, the material presented is descriptive rather than prescriptive and no responsibility for its implementation is to be assumed by author or publisher.

Chapter 10 explores the psychotherapeutic approaches of dynamic and cognitive-behavioral strategies. The substantive descriptions and sample interactions will serve as an organizational guide as you develop your professional procedures.

The final two chapters deal with discussions of fringe benefits and retirement, and what being an expert witness entails. A discussion of the interplay between the mental health and legal professions, although recognized as an important issue, rarely finds its way into books that deal with independent practice. Chapter 11, "On Being an Expert Witness" presents an in-depth discussion of what the clinician can expect when going from subpoena to the witness stand. The closing chapter provides invaluable aid in managing the financial rewards of successful practice.

There are many clinicians, researchers, publishers, and friends to whom I am deeply grateful for encouragement, support, and help provided in bringing this book to fruition. I am pleased to acknowledge permission to quote or reproduce various copyrighted works. The following materials are presented in detail in the text:

*Code of Ethics for Social Workers,* rev. ed., copyright 1979. Reprinted with permission of the National Association for Social Workers.

*Specialty Guidelines for the Delivery of Services by Clinical Psychologists,* copyright 1981, and "Principles of Confidentiality" from *Ethical Standards for Psychologists,* copyright 1977 by The American Psychological Association and printed with permission of the publisher.

Financial worksheets adapted from *Establishing and Maintaining a Successful and Independent Practice,* by Mark Lewin, copyright 1978 by Professional Development Group, Upstate Psychological Service Center, and printed with permission of the publisher and author.

Special points relevant to newsprint from *The Scientist's Responsibility for Public Information* by Neal Miller, copyright 1978 by the Society for Neuroscience and printed with permission of the publisher.

The cover page from the *Wechsler Intelligence Scale for Children—Revised,* copyright 1971, 1974, all rights reserved, by The Psychological Corporation, New York, N.Y., and reprinted with permission.

"Reporting Psychological Test Results to Patients and Their Families," by J. Richman, *Journal of Projective Techniques and Personality Assessment,* June 1974, copyright 1974 by the Society for Personality Assessment and printed with permission of the publisher and author.

Tables describing chemotherapy from *A Manual for Clinical Psychologists,* by James Choca, copyright 1980 by James Choca and printed with permission of the author and publisher, Brunner/Mazel, Inc.

Sections adapted from Chapter 11, "Pharmacotherapy," from *Human Resources for Troubled Children,* by Werner I. Halpern and Stanley Kissel, copyright 1976 by John Wiley & Sons, Inc. and reprinted with permission of the publisher and authors.

Sections from "A Thought Stopping Procedure," by J. R. Cautela and P. A. Wisocki, *The Psychological Record*, 1977; copyright 1977 by *The Psychological Record* and reprinted with permission of the publisher and authors.

Glossary of Legal Terms, reprinted with permission from *The Psychologist as Expert Witness,* 1964, pp. 2–9, by Harold Liebenson and Joseph Wepman. Published by Callaghan & Company, 3201 Old Glenview Road, Wilmette, Illinois 60091, printed with permission of the publisher.

Portions of *Outline for Psychiatric Examination,* by S. Mouchly Small, copyright 1978 by Sandoz and printed with permission of the author and publisher.

The foresight of the Panorama Pediatric Group provided a laboratory for many of the ideas expressed throughout this book.

I am most appreciative of the support during this work of the Rochester Mental Health Center and especially Dr. Werner I. Halpern, Director of the Children and Youth Division. Thanks are also due to Barbara Beard and Cindy Deane for their assistance in typing the manuscript.

Finally, I want to express a special thanks to R. Curtis Whitesel, who until his untimely death, was editorial director of Aspen Systems. His confidence, encouragement, and the many helpful comments and suggestions he made throughout the completion of this book are testimony to dedicated and responsible publishing expertise.

*Stanley Kissel, Ph.D.*
March 1983

Chapter 1

# Know Thy Professional Self

# 1

Early in my professional career, a friend who was in the independent practice of accounting invited me to a cocktail party with the advice, "Mingle and make contacts." At the party, he continually brought the conversation around to business, economics, and the importance of knowing how to manage one's money for investment and tax purposes. I was surprised by these tactics but recognized that he was quite a businessman. When we spoke afterwards, he told me "Marketing is the name of the game." I thought to myself rather smugly that I did not have to play that game; I was able to keep business and profession separate. My reasoning went something like this: If I wanted to be a businessman, I would have gone into business. I wanted to be a professional, and thus I chose a profession.

Many of my colleagues shared this view. I received much consentient validation from people I spoke with and also from those in other professions. At the time there were very strict and stringent rules regarding advertisements, announcements, and promotional materials.

The recent emerging literature on independent practice has swung to the other extreme, suggesting that the practitioner, independent or publicly based, is very much "in business" and the product is the clinical work he or she is engaged in.

Most mental health practitioners, such as clinical psychologists, social workers, marriage therapists, psychiatric nurses, guidance counselors, school psychologists, vocational psychologists, and drug counselors, go into their chosen professions for reasons that, although quite diverse, often have in common their dislike for business and business-related enterprises. Indeed, when many practitioners find themselves face to face with the business aspects of their practice they become very uncomfortable. Such a response is quite understandable. They have generally been poorly prepared for this aspect of their profession. Full-time independent practitioners attempt to resolve this dilemma by hiring "tough business managers" to handle the nonclinical aspects of their practice. Part-time practitioners' business dilemmas are somewhat different, although they are philosophically and attitudinally in the same boat. They find themselves with similar feelings regarding the business aspects of their practice, yet part of the time they are engaged in the public practice of their chosen profession—with a steady income that can be a dual-edge sword. On one side it provides a cushion of security and on the other, ready-made rationalizations for sloppy approaches to the business demands of their practice.

When I began to practice part time on a private basis in Rochester, New York, the average fee was $25.00 a visit. I had the rent-free use of a colleague's office; thus I reasoned my "overhead" was zero. When I met with a couple for my first private appointment, I set a fee of $15.00 an hour, justifying the very low fee on the basis of the aforementioned low overhead. In addition, I told myself that this was not an important source of income for me. I was guided by such lofty views as: "The money I receive will pay only for luxuries," and "The family I am seeing might not be as economically fortunate as I." As quick as I had a summary conference with the couple, made some suggestions based upon my evaluation, and had some feedback from the referral source saying that the couple was pleased with my services, my professional fees increased. The second case I saw was billed at $25.00 a visit. It was clear that my rationale of low overhead, limited need for extra income, guilt about luxuries, and pseudoaltruism concerning my patients' economic well-being were all rationalizations to help with my own concerns regarding independent practice.

It is important for the professional who contemplates independent practice, whether part time or full time, to become cognizant of and thus avoid the underlying business minimization trap. The practitioner must recognize and respect the importance of the business aspects of independent practice. Note, I said "business aspects," which does not mean that the practitioner is or has to be a business person. However, the practitioner must acknowledge the fact that there are elements of business—billing, collection, record keeping, marketing—that are definite requirements for the development and maintenance of a successful practice.

Perceiving oneself as a professional, not a business person, heightens interest in the conceptual and clinical end of the practice. The practitioner understandably expresses more concern about models of intervention, appropriate diagnostic tools, and tactics for helping troubled and at times troublesome clients. Essentially, many practitioners characterize the choice as business versus profession. It is no secret which side of the dichotomy most professionals choose. They have been indoctrinated by teachers whose philosophy embodies the scientific quest for knowledge and clinical methods regardless of time, cost, or efficiency. However, rather than embrace one to the exclusion of the other, the practitioner would do well to consider each a separate side of the same coin, and both leading to growth in providing professional services to a needy clientele.

Indeed, it is clear that more and more people are turning to psychologists and other nonmedical practitioners for solutions to their emotional misery and problems of coping with life stresses. The past two decades have seen an increasing concern, almost a preoccupation, with psychological ailments and psychological well-being. Loneliness, alienation, communication speedups have all been indicted as major stresses of the modern individual. Such slogans as "getting it all together," "letting it all hang loose," and "better living through chemistry" have come to symbolize the need for professional help from a variety of human service providers. The rise in delinquency, the greater utilization of hospital beds by patients suffering from mental and emotional disorders, and the alarming rate increase of behavior and learning problems in schools are just some indications of the need for mental health practitioners. While many families seek out such help from community centers, family courts, town counseling services, family service agencies, and mental health centers, a growing majority are looking more and more toward the private sector, where they feel they have more control in choosing the professional they will be seeing.

Although professionals feel well equipped to provide such services in the confines of the public sphere, they often find themselves ill equipped and ill prepared for independent practice. Their limitations are usually not in the realm of knowing how to determine what ails their clients or how to go about providing assistance using accepted procedures. The problem is in areas that are not difficult to remedy, if only there is the inclination and desire. For example, most clinical psychologists' formal training is in the scientific area. The model that guided my education was labeled the Boulder model. The model emerged from a training director's meeting held in Boulder, Colorado and suggested that a clinical psychologist provides clinical services, teaches, and does scientific research. There is an underlying attitude of modesty regarding accomplishment, not only in talking with clients but also with the public at large. "A low profile is a good profile" might be an apt slogan for this orientation. Such an approach to some extent has to be renounced by the independent practitioner if he or she is to be successful. The independent practitioner must pay attention to three major areas: attitudinal, conceptual, and ethical.

## ATTITUDINAL CONSIDERATIONS

Successful practitioners advise those embarking on independent practice to give serious consideration to the special stresses involved in such practice and their personal strengths for coping with them. The following discussion of attitudinal considerations is not presented as exhaustive but includes those ideas most emphasized by successful practitioners (Harrower, 1961; Lewin, 1978; and Pressman, 1979).

## Uncertainty

The self-employed practitioner faces the major uncertainty in the realm of income. This is especially true while establishing the practice. The type and amount of uncertainty, of course, will vary, depending on whether the practitioner embarks on full time or part time practice. Harrower (1961) suggested that beginners "keep your full time job and put in a few evenings a week seeing your own patients" (p. 7). Pressman (1979) has found that a full-time practitioner would need to schedule 22 clients a week at $45.00/clinical hour to gross a weekly income of $800.00, which is adjusted for cancellations and poor collections. Of course, the lower the hourly rate, the greater the number of interviews necessary to obtain the same gross weekly income. Pressman estimates that a full-time practitioner can expect to achieve a level of 22 scheduled appointments a week within approximately one year's time. Remember your gross income shrinks as a result of fixed and variable overhead, government taxes, and social security. More will be said about these expenses in the next chapter.

There is no monthly paycheck. Thus the psychologist or other mental health practitioner in private practice needs to be sufficiently disciplined in the management of funds—both personal and business—to accommodate the peaks and valleys of independent practice.

The part-time practitioner who plans to combine public and private practice can count on some steady income. The uncertainty for the part-timer involves the often nebulous issue, conflict of interest. Referring patients seen at a public facility to yourself is a conflict of interest and should be avoided. However, there are a multitude of other practices, such as speaking with private patients while in the pay of a public facility or writing up notes about your private patients during free time in your public facility, where the issue is not so clear cut.

There are situations where working in a public sector can be helpful to the practitioner's private practice without causing a conflict of interest. We will consider this in greater detail in Chapter 5.

## Contact with Other Professionals

Another major consideration is how strong a need one has for interpersonal stimulation, that is, contacts with other professionals during the work day.

The need for chitchat, consentient validation of ideas, or just another member to work with as a team should be considered. The professional who functions in a community mental health center with other professionals has the luxury of consulting with colleagues regarding knotty problems or testing out his or her own point of view. Indeed, it is not uncommon for practitioners working at a community mental health center or county clinic to schedule time on a regular basis for contacts with supervisory personnel for just such purposes. Little concern is often given to the cost of such time. However, the private practitioner is not only geographically separated from his or her colleagues but is constantly mindful of the fact that "time is money."

This adage can also cloud the independent practitioner's mind to the need for refurbishing skills, keeping up with changes in the field, or even gaining new skills. A survey of state psychological examining boards revealed that nine states currently have a continuing education plan: Colorado, Iowa, Maryland, New Mexico, Oregon, Texas, Utah, Washington, and West Virginia. (APA monitor, April, 1981). The specific number of continuing education hours required for recertification or relicensing varies from ten hours over a two-year period in West Virginia to one hundred and fifty hours over a three-year period in Washington, but the average seems to be around twenty-five a year. Seventeen additional states are currently at different stages in their continuing education requirements: Alabama, Alaska, Arkansas, California, Delaware, Kansas, Louisiana, Massachusetts, Michigan, Minnesota, Mississippi, Nevada, New Hampshire, North Carolina, Rhode Island, Vermont, and Wyoming. Nineteen states have mandatory continuing education programs in psychiatry: Alaska, Arizona, California, Colorado, Hawaii, Illinois, Iowa, Kansas, Maryland, Massachusetts, Michigan, Minnesota, New Hampshire, New Mexico, Ohio, Rhode Island, Utah, Washington, and Wisconsin. Currently, only California has continuing education requirements for social workers. (APA Monitor, April, 1981)

Another area affected by the independent practitioner's financial concerns involves vacations. Often minimized or at times overlooked is the need for recharging personal batteries.

## Administration and Organization

Such mundane tasks as scheduling appointments, billing, sending out statements, keeping and organizing records are provided free of "conceptual headache" to the professional who works in a public agency. Administrators, secretaries, and receptionists are all there to serve his or her needs. The independent practitioner must devote time to these tasks, for which, as we have seen, there has often been little training or interest. The successful full-time practitioner may have the luxury of hiring "a girl Friday" to execute these tasks, yet time will still have to be allocated for developing and overseeing the system.

The part-time practitioner and clinician just getting started will not have the luxury of a paid administrator or office manager. Keep in mind the caveat that when one becomes sloppy with office work, it spills over into clinical practice. This is clearly evident when working with children. Although you may have a perfectly good working relationship with the child, if animosity over administrative business such as billing develops with the parents, the child can get caught in the middle.

### Initiative

Recall the accountant at the cocktail party who was constantly "on the make for new business." He did not shy away from opportunities to initiate possible new referral sources. Many mental health practitioners engaged in practice in the public sector view themselves as behavioral scientists, researchers, or "professionals" and shy away from marketing themselves or their skills. Like it or not, the public makes little distinction between the person and the skill. Your attitude toward presenting yourself positively, and at times seemingly immodestly, becomes an aspect of marketing. More about this in Chapters 4 and 5.

### Follow-Through

Consider for a moment the fact that many large institutionalized mental health agencies have "tickler systems" built in to remind the professional to perform certain chores. For example, at the Children's Division of the Rochester Mental Health Center, at the conclusion of a diagnostic evaluation, usually ending with a parent conference, the secretary reminds the appropriate staff to send out a follow-up note to the referral source. A reasonable expectation, reporting back to the referral source, was being neglected by competent professionally trained clinical staff until the introduction of the tickler.

Who will remind you in private practice that you neglected to get back to the referral source? The follow-through on such commitments as sending out reports on time, or returning phone calls within a reasonable period of time, is a necessary consideration for initiating and continuing successful private practice.

### Stress Tolerance

The mental health practitioner is in a stressful occupation. When the practitioner serves in the public domain the support systems of his or her colleagues and the entire agency are available. In independent practice the professional is alone. The constant concern about referrals, cash flow, competition, and family obligations, not to mention the myriad clinical decisions that have to be made daily, clearly tax even those with high stress tolerance. Burnout, that is, depleting oneself physically and mentally, has become a particular hazard in the helping professions. Private practitioners appear to be at even greater risk for this occupational malady than their professional colleagues employed by the public sector. A major cause of burnout is a mismatch between outcome and effort. Helping disturbed and needy people is very difficult! The advice to separate work from the rest of life is often difficult for those mental health specialists who practice independently.

### Salesmanship

The independent practitioner is constantly selling and has to be alert to opportunities to further advance the practice. In addition, you have to be aware of the personal impact you have on people. Do you come across as strong, decisive, soft, casual, quiet, or timid?

Practicing in one sphere, the hard sell might be an asset, while in another a liability—to be able to gauge your impact is an important aspect of the ultimately successful private practitioner.

The attitudinal aspects we have examined involve management and organizational inclinations, personality and self-motivation traits, and marketing propensities. If you find yourself reacting more unfavorably than favorably, especially in the realm of marketing, then perhaps your temperament is not suited for private practice.

## CONCEPTUAL SKILLS

Most clinicians contemplating independent practice may take the conceptual aspect of their work—namely, that of being a skilled and competent practitioner—for granted. Knowing what is in your head is one thing; communicating it to clients who are anxious and do not speak your language is another matter. A person can be an expert on personality theory (with many publications to your credit) and an excellent diagnostician, and still be a poor practitioner and in need of supervision.

You will have to give careful consideration to the type of service or services you will provide to the public. Will you limit your practice to children, adolescents, adults, or will you see clients of any age?

Will you view yourself as capable of helping people of all levels of pathology—an autistic child; an adolescent in turmoil; a neurotic housewife; an assaultive, unemployed 40-year-old; a delusional schizophrenic? Will you limit your expertise to "neurotic complaints"?

Will your practice be exclusively devoted to diagnostic work or will you strive to become known exclusively as a psychotherapist?

Will you be guided by one conceptual schema to the exclusion of others such as behavior modification, biofeedback, hypnotism, group therapy, or family therapy? Are you interested in becoming a "professional's" professional and providing supervision to other independent practitioners? Do you see yourself as becoming affiliated with other practitioners, both medical and nonmedical, whose services can complement your own so as to provide a full range of service?

The manner in which you conceptualize your skills will impact both on the way you market yourself and the type of office facilities you will choose. The practitioner who devotes much time to family therapy will furnish his or her office quite differently than a clinician doing predominantly play therapy. While the former may attempt to simulate the comfort of a living room with some oversized chairs and possibly a couch, the latter would want quarters where concerns about spillage and breakage would be minimized.

It is extremely important for you to consider your level of expertise prior to "putting out a shingle." More space will be devoted to this issue as it is as much an ethical as a competence issue.

How you convey information to clients and referral sources will stem from your conceptual understanding of health and pathology, your theoretical orientation, and the way in which you organize your information and material.

Whether you are form oriented or talk oriented, how you feed back your information will have profound ramifications for your continued success as an independent practitioner. We will delve into this important area in Chapters 5 and 6.

## ETHICS

Human service providers are neither equally comfortable in nor equally qualified for providing clinical services to the public for a fee. Unfortunately, many in the helping services see themselves as ready to provide help and function as independent practitioners. Some of these have proper academic *credentials,* but their training is scholarly and not professional. There is a world of difference between one who knows and one who does; between a scientific researcher, a clinical psychologist, and a competent professional practitioner. Furthermore, there are also levels of training and competency: a master's degree psychologist or social worker, a graduate from a human services program, a drug counselor with two years on-the-job training, a psychiatrist completing the residency, an MSW state-certified social worker, or a Ph.D. psychologist with a diplomate. Most professions, such as psychiatry, social work, and psychology, have codes of ethics and standards of practice that are shared by all members. These codes provide guidance to clinicians considering whether or not they are ready for independent practice. Clinicians from areas that do not have professional allegiance to one of these three professions would do well to familiarize themselves with some of these professional standards for practice.

Members of the National Association of Social Workers subscribe to such a code of ethics as a basis for professional conduct and agree to submit to the adjudication of grievance procedures of the Association. Those listed in the register who are not NASW members but who hold a state license at a level at least equivalent to the autonomous practice standards of the Academy of Certified Social Workers are bound by the adjudication procedures incorporated in their state licensing law (NASW Register of Clinical Social Workers, 1978).

A summary of the code of ethics that social workers subscribe to is presented in Exhibit 1–1.

---

**Exhibit 1–1** Social Work Code of Ethics

I. *The Social Worker's Conduct and Comportment as a Social Worker*

A. Propriety. The social worker should maintain high standards of personal conduct in the capacity of identity as social worker.

B. Competence and Professional Development. The social worker should strive to become and remain proficient in professional practice and the performance of professional functions.

C. Service. The social worker should regard as primary the service obligation of the social work profession.

D. Integrity. The social worker should act in accordance with the highest standards of professional integrity.

E. Scholarship and Research. The social worker engaged in study and research should be guided by the conventions of scholarly inquiry.

II. *The Social Worker's Ethical Responsibility to Clients*

F. Primacy of Clients' Interests. The social worker's primary responsibility is to clients.

*(continues)*

**Exhibit 1–1** continued

G. Rights and Prerogatives of Clients. The social worker should make every effort to foster maximum self-determination on the part of clients.

H. Confidentiality and Privacy. The social worker should respect the privacy of clients and hold in confidence all information obtained in the course of professional service.

I. Fees. When setting fees, the social worker should ensure that they are fair, reasonable, considerate, and commensurate with the service performed and with due regard for the clients' ability to pay.

III. *The Social Worker's Ethical Responsibility to Colleagues*

J. Respect, Fairness, and Courtesy. The social worker should treat colleagues with respect, courtesy, fairness, and good faith.

K. Dealing with Colleagues' Clients. The social worker has the responsibility to relate to the clients of colleagues with full professional consideration.

IV. *The Social Worker's Ethical Responsibility to Employers and Employing Organizations*

L. Commitments to Employing Organizations. The social worker should adhere to commitments made to the employing organizations.

V. *The Social Worker's Ethical Responsibility to the Social Work Profession*

M. Maintaining the Integrity of the Profession. The social worker should uphold and advance the values, ethics, knowledge, and mission of the profession.

N. Community Service. The social worker should assist the profession in making social services available to the general public.

O. Development of Knowledge. The social worker should take responsibility for identifying, developing, and fully utilizing knowledge for professional practice.

VI. *The Social Worker's Ethical Responsibility to Society*

P. Promoting the General Welfare. The social worker should promote the general welfare of society.

As a member of the National Association of Social Workers I commit myself to conduct my professional relationships in accord with the code and subscribe to the following statements:

I regard as my primary obligation the welfare of the individual or group serviced, which includes action for improving social conditions.

I will not discriminate because of race, color, religion, age, sex or national ancestry and in my job capacity will work to prevent and eliminate such discrimination in rendering service, in work assignments, and in employment practices.

I give precedence to my professional responsibility over my personal interests.

I hold myself responsible for the quality and extent of the service I perform.

I respect the privacy of the people I serve.

I use in a responsible manner information gained in professional relationships.

I treat with respect the findings, views, and actions of colleagues and use appropriate channels to express judgment on these matters.

I practice social work within the recognized knowledge and competence of the profession.

**Exhibit 1–1** continued

I recognize my professional responsibility to add my ideas and findings to the body of social work knowledge and practice.

I accept responsibility to help protect the community against unethical practice by any individuals or organizations engaged in social welfare activities.

I stand ready to give appropriate professional service in public emergencies.

I distinguish clearly, in public, between my statements and actions as an individual and as a representative of an organization.

I support the principle that professional practice requires professional education.

I accept responsibility for working toward the creation and maintenance of conditions within agencies that enable social workers to conduct themselves in keeping with this code.

I contribute my knowledge, skills, and support to programs of human welfare.

*Source:* Published 1979, National Association of Social Workers, Inc. Reprinted with permission, from *Professional Standards*, Washington, DC: Professions NASW, 1980.

Although all members of the American Psychological Association also subscribe to a code of ethics, the Association encompasses a divergent membership whose interests range from examining the reactions of a rat's brain to engaging in the independent practice of clinical psychology. In addition to its code of ethics, the American Psychological Association has also designed standards for the delivery of psychological services by clinical psychologists. These are presented in Exhibit 1–2 along with references following the guidelines.

These codes do not guarantee ethical conduct but they at least guarantee that the practitioner has considered his or her level of competency and provided the public with procedures that can lead to censure by the profession. In addition, a number of states have legal requirements governing the use of various titles for the rendering of services to the public. Every state in the Union requires physicians to be licensed but there are no requirements that they have to be board certified in psychiatry to practice as psychiatrists. Forty-four states require that psychologists be either licensed or certified and twenty-two states require the same for social workers.

In many states it is just the title "psychologist" or "social worker" that is restricted. Professionals can provide services using the techniques of social work, psychiatry, or psychology, while calling themselves "psychotherapists" or "counselors." The legal regulations for the practice of mental health by the subspecialties are minimal and thus place a great burden on the individual practitioner and the professional associations.

**Exhibit 1–2** Specialty Guidelines for the Delivery of Services by Clinical Psychologists

Guideline 1

PROVIDERS

1.1 Each clinical psychological service unit offering psychological services has available at least one professional clinical psychologist and as many more professional clinical psychologists as are necessary to assure the adequacy and quality of services offered.

INTERPRETATION: The intent of this Guideline is that one or more providers of psychological services in any clinical psychological service unit meet the levels of training and experience of the professional clinical psychologist as specified in the preceding definitions.

When a facility offering clinical psychological services does not have a full time professional clinical psychologist available, the facility retains the services of one or more professional clinical psychologists on a regular part time basis. The clinical psychologist so retained directs and supervises the psychological services provided, participates sufficiently to be able to assess the need for services, reviews the content of services provided, and has the authority to assume professional responsibility and accountability for them.

The psychologist directing the service unit is responsible for determining and justifying appropriate ratios of psychologists to users and psychologists to support staff, in order to ensure proper scope, accessibility, and quality of services provided in that setting.

1.2 Providers of clinical psychological services who do not meet the requirements for the professional clinical psychologist are supervised directly by a professional clinical psychologist who assumes professional responsibility and accountability for the services provided. The level and extent of supervision may vary from task to task so long as the supervising psychologist retains a sufficiently close supervisory relationship to meet this Guideline. Special proficiency training or supervision may be provided by a professional psychologist of another speciality or by a professional from another discipline whose competence in the given area has been demonstrated by previous training and experience.

INTERPRETATION: In each clinical psychological service unit there may be varying levels of responsibility with respect to the nature and quality of services provided. Support personnel are considered to be responsible for their functions and behavior when assisting in the provision of clinical psychological services and are accountable to the professional clinical psychologist. Ultimate professional responsibility and accountability for the services provided require that the supervisor review and approve reports and test protocols, review and approve intervention plans and strategies, and review outcomes. Therefore, the supervision of all clinical psychological services is provided directly by a professional clinical psychologist in individual and/or group face-to-face meetings.

In order to meet this Guideline, an appropriate number of hours per week are devoted to direct face-to-face supervision of each clinical psychological service unit staff member. In no event is such supervision less than 1 hour per week. The more comprehensive the psychological services are, the more supervision is needed. A plan or formula for relating increasing amounts of supervisory time to the complexity of professional responsibilities is to be developed. The amount and nature of supervision is made known to all parties concerned.

**Exhibit 1–2** continued

Such communications are in writing and describe and delineate the duties of the employee with respect to range and type of services to be provided. The limits of independent action and decision making are defined. The description of responsibility also specifies the means by which the employee will contact the professional clinical psychologist in the event of emergency or crisis situations.

1.3 Wherever a clinical psychological service unit exists, a professional clinical psychologist is responsible for planning, directing, and reviewing the provision of clinical psychological services. Whenever the clinical psychological service unit is part of a larger professional psychological service encompassing various psychological specialties, a professional psychologist is the administrative head of the service.

INTERPRETATION: The clinical psychologist coordinates the activities of the clinical psychological service unit with other professional, administrative, and technical groups, both within and outside the facility. This clinical psychologist, who may be the director, chief, or coordinator of the clinical psychological service unit, has related responsibilities including, but not limited to, recruiting qualified staff, directing training and research activities of the service, maintaining a high level of professional and ethical practice, and ensuring that staff members function only within the areas of their competency.

To facilitate the effectiveness of clinical services by raising the level of staff sensitivity and professional skills, the clinical psychologist designated as director is responsible for participating in the selection of staff and support personnel whose qualifications and skills (e.g., language, cultural and experiential background, race, sex, and age) are directly relevant to the needs and characteristics of the users served.

1.4 When functioning as part of an organizational setting, professional clinical psychologists bring their backgrounds and skills to bear on the goals of the organization, whenever appropriate, by participation in the planning and development of overall services.

INTERPRETATION: Professional clinical psychologists participate in the maintenance of high professional standards by representation on committees concerned with service delivery.

As appropriate to the setting, their activities may include active participation, as voting and as office-holding members, on the professional staffs of hospitals and other facilities and on other executive, planning, and evaluation boards and committees.

1.5 Clinical psychologists maintain current knowledge of scientific and professional developments to preserve and enhance their professional competence.

INTERPRETATION: Methods through which knowledge of scientific and professional developments may be gained include, but are not limited to, reading scientific and professional publications, attendance at workshops, participation in staff development programs, and other forms of continuing education. The clinical psychologist has ready access to reference material related to the provision of psychological services. Clinical psychologists are prepared to show evidence periodically that they are staying abreast of current knowledge and practices in the field of clinical psychology through continuing education.

1.6 Clinical psychologists limit their practice to their demonstrated areas of professional competence.

INTERPRETATION: Clinical psychological services are offered in accordance with the providers' areas of competence as defined by verifiable training and experience. When extending services beyond the range of their usual practice, psychologists obtain pertinent training or

*(continues)*

**Exhibit 1–2** continued

appropriate professional supervision. Such training or supervision is consistent with the extension of functions performed and services provided. An extension of services may involve a change in the theoretical orientation of the clinical psychologist, a change in modality or technique, or a change in the type of client and/or the kinds of problems or disorders for which services are to be provided (e.g., children, elderly persons, mental retardation, neurological impairment).

1.7 Professional psychologists who wish to qualify as clinical psychologists meet the same requirements with respect to subject matter and professional skills that apply to doctoral and postdoctoral education and training in clinical psychology.

INTERPRETATION: Education of doctoral-level psychologists to qualify them for specialty practice in clinical psychology is under the auspices of a department in a regionally accredited university or of a professional school that offers the doctoral degree in clinical psychology. Such education is individualized, with due credit being given for relevant course work and other requirements that have previously been satisfied. In addition, doctoral-level training plus 1 year of postdoctoral experience supervised by a clinical psychologist is required. Merely taking an internship in clinical psychology or acquiring experience in a practicum setting is not adequate preparation for becoming a clinical psychologist when prior education has not been in that area. Fulfillment of such an individualized educational program is attested to by the awarding of a certificate by the supervising department or professional school that indicates the successful completion of preparation in clinical psychology.

1.8 Professional clinical psychologists are encouraged to develop innovative theories and procedures and to provide appropriate theoretical and/or empirical support for their innovations.

INTERPRETATION: A specialty of a profession rooted in a science intends continually to explore and experiment with a view to developing and verifying new and improved methods of serving the public in ways that can be documented.

Guideline 2

PROGRAMS

2.1 Composition and organization of a clinical psychological service unit:

2.1.1 The composition and programs of a clinical psychological service unit are responsive to the needs of the persons or setting served.

INTERPRETATION: A clinical psychological service unit is structured so as to facilitate effective and economical delivery of services. For example, a clinical psychological service unit serving predominantly a low-income, ethnic, or racial minority group has a staffing pattern and service programs that are adapted to the linguistic, experiential, and attitudinal characteristics of the users.

2.1.2 A description of the organization of the clinical psychological service unit and its lines of responsibility and accountability for the delivery of psychological services is available in written form to staff of the unit and to users and sanctioners upon request.

INTERPRETATION: The description includes lines of responsibility, supervisory relationships, and the level and extent of accountability for each person who provides psychological services.

2.1.3 A clinical psychological service unit includes sufficient numbers of professional and support personnel to achieve its goals, objectives, and purposes.

INTERPRETATION: The work load and diversity of psychological services required and the specific goals and objectives of the setting determine the numbers and qualifications of

**Exhibit 1–2** continued

professional and support personnel in the clinical psychological service unit. Where shortages in personnel exist, so that psychological services cannot be rendered in a professional manner, the director of the clinical psychological service unit initiates action to remedy such shortages. When this fails, the director appropriately modifies the scope or work load of the unit to maintain the quality of the services rendered.

2.2 Policies:

2.2.1 When the clinical psychological service unit is composed of more than one person or is a component of a larger organization, a written statement of its objectives and scope of services is developed, maintained, and reviewed.

INTERPRETATION: The clinical psychological service unit reviews its objectives and scope of services annually and revises them as necessary to ensure that the psychological services offered are consistent with staff competencies and current psychological knowledge and practice. This statement is discussed with staff, reviewed with the appropriate administrator, and distributed to users and sanctioners upon request, whenever appropriate.

2.2.2 All providers within a clinical psychological service unit support the legal and civil rights of the users.

INTERPRETATION: Providers of clinical psychological services safeguard the interests of the users with regard to personal, legal, and civil rights. They are continually sensitive to the issue of confidentiality of information, the short term and long term impacts of their decision and recommendations, and other matters pertaining to individual, legal, and civil rights. Concerns regarding the safeguarding of individual rights of users include, but are not limited to, problems of self-incrimination in judicial proceedings, involuntary commitment to hospitals, protection of minors or legal incompetents, discriminatory practices in employment selection procedures, recommendations for special education provisions, information relative to adverse personnel actions in the armed services, and adjudication of domestic relations disputes in divorce and custodial proceedings. Providers of clinical psychological services take affirmative action by making themselves available to local committees, review boards, and similar advisory groups established to safeguard the human, civil, and legal rights of service users.

2.2.3 All providers within a clinical psychological service unit are familiar with and adhere to the American Psychological Association's Standards for Providers of Psychological Services, Ethical Principles of Psychologists, Standards for Educational and Psychological Tests, Ethical Principles in the Conduct of Research With Human Participants, and other official policy statements relevant to standards for professional services issued by the Association.

INTERPRETATION: Providers of clinical psychological services maintain up-to-date knowledge of the relevant standards of the American Psychological Association.

2.2.4 All providers within a clinical and psychological service unit conform to relevant statutes established by federal, state, and local governments.

INTERPRETATION: All providers of clinical psychological services are familiar with appropriate statutes regulating the practice of psychology. They observe agency regulations that have the force of law and that relate to the delivery of psychological services (e.g., evaluation for disability retirement and special education placements). In addition, all providers are cognizant that federal agencies such as the Veterans Administration, the Department of Education, and the Department of Health and Human Services have policy statements regarding psychological services, and where relevant, providers conform to them. Providers

*(continues)*

**Exhibit 1–2** continued

of clinical psychological services are also familiar with other statutes and regulations, including those addressed to the civil and legal rights of users (e.g., those promulgated by the federal Equal Employment Opportunity Commission), that are pertinent to their scope of practice.

It is the responsibility of the American Psychological Association to maintain current files of those federal policies, statutes, and regulations relating to this section and to assist its members in obtaining them. The state psychological associations and the state licensing boards periodically publish and distribute appropriate state statutes and regulations.

2.2.5 All providers within a clinical psychological service unit inform themselves about and use the network of human services in their communities in order to link users with relevant services and resources.

INTERPRETATION: Clinical psychologists and support staff are sensitive to the broader context of human needs. In recognizing the matrix of personal and societal problems, providers make available to users information regarding human services such as legal aid societies, social services, employment agencies, health resources, and educational and recreational facilities. Providers of clinical psychological services refer to such community resources and, when indicated, actively intervene on behalf of the users.

Community resources include the private as well as the public sectors. Private resources include private agencies and centers and psychologists in independent private practice. Consultation is sought or referral made within the public or private network of services whenever required in the best interest of the users. Clinical psychologists, in either the private or the public setting, utilize other resources in the community whenever indicated because of limitations within the psychological service unit providing the services. Professional clinical psychologists in private practice are familiar with the types of services offered through local community mental health clinics and centers, including alternatives to hospitalization, and know the costs and eligibility requirements for those services.

2.2.6 In the delivery of clinical psychological services, the providers maintain a cooperative relationship with colleagues and co-workers in the best interest of the users.

INTERPRETATION: Clinical psychologists recognize the areas of special competence of other professional psychologists and of professionals in other fields for either consultation or referral purposes. Providers of clinical psychological services make appropriate use of other professional, research, technical, and administrative resources to serve the best interests of users and establish and maintain cooperative arrangements with such other resources as required to meet the needs of users.

2.3 Procedures:

2.3.1 Each clinical psychological service unit follows a set of procedural guidelines for the delivery of psychological services.

INTERPRETATION: Providers are prepared to provide a statement of procedural guidelines, in either oral or written form, in terms that can be understood by users, including sanctioners and local administrators. This statement describes the current methods, forms, procedures, and techniques being used to achieve the objectives and goals for psychological services.

2.3.2 Providers of clinical psychological services develop plans appropriate to the providers' professional practices and to the problems presented by the users.

INTERPRETATION: A clinical psychologist develops a plan that describes the psychological services, their objectives, and the manner in which they will be provided. This plan is in written form; it serves as a basis for obtaining understanding and concurrence from the users and provides a mechanism for subsequent peer review. This plan is, of course, modified as new needs or information develop.

**Exhibit 1–2** continued

A clinical psychologist who provides services as one member of a collaborative effort participates in the development and implementation of the overall service plan and provides for its periodic review.

2.3.3 Accurate, current, and pertinent documentation of essential clinical psychological services provided is maintained.

INTERPRETATION: Records kept of clinical psychological services may include, but are not limited to, identifying data, dates of services, types of services, significant actions taken, and outcome at termination. Providers of clinical psychological services ensure that essential information concerning services rendered is recorded within a reasonable time following their completion.

2.3.4 Each clinical psychological service unit follows an established record retention and disposition policy.

INTERPRETATION: The policy on record retention and disposition conforms to federal or state statutes or administrative regulations where such are applicable. In the absence of such regulations, the policy is (a) that the full record be retained intact for 3 years after the completion of planned services or after the date of last contact with the user, whichever is later; (b) that a full record or summary of the record be maintained for an additional 12 years; and (c) that the record may be disposed of no sooner than 15 years after the completion of planned services or after the date of the last contact, whichever is later. These temporal guides are consistent with procedures currently in use by federal record centers.

In the event of the death or incapacity of a clinical psychologist in independent practice, special procedures are necessary to ensure the continuity of active services to users and the proper safeguarding of inactive records being retained to meet this Guideline. Following approval by the affected user, it is appropriate for another clinical psychologist, acting under the auspices of the local professional standards review committee (PSRC), to review the records with the user and recommend a course of action for continuing professional service, if needed. Depending on local circumstances, the reviewing psychologist may also recommend appropriate arrangements for the balance of the record retention and disposition period.

This Guideline has been designed to meet a variety of circumstances that may arise, often years after a set of psychological services has been completed. More and more records are being used in forensic matters, for peer review, and in response to requests from users, other professionals, or other legitimate parties requiring accurate information about the exact dates, nature, course, and outcome of a set of psychological services. These record retention procedures also provide valuable baseline data for the original psychologist-provider when a previous user returns for additional services.

2.3.5 Providers of clinical psychological services maintain a system to protect confidentiality of their records.

INTERPRETATION: Clinical psychologists are responsible for maintaining the confidentiality of information about users of services, from whatever source derived. All persons supervised by clinical psychologists, including nonprofessional personnel and students, who have access to records of psychological services are required to maintain this confidentiality as a condition of employment.

The clinical psychologist does not release confidential information, except with the written consent of the user directly involved or his or her legal representative. Even after consent for

*(continues)*

**Exhibit 1–2** continued

release has been obtained, the clinical psychologist clearly identifies such information as confidential to the recipient of the information. If directed otherwise by statute or regulations with the force of law or by court order, the psychologist may seek a resolution to the conflict that is both ethically and legally feasible and appropriate.

Users are informed in advance of any limits in the setting for maintenance of confidentiality of psychological information. For instance, clinical psychologists in hospital, clinic, or agency settings inform their patients that psychological information in a patient's clinical record may be available without the patient's written consent to other members of the professional staff associated with the patient's treatment or rehabilitation. Similar limitations on confidentiality of psychological information may be present in certain school, industrial, military, or other institutional settings, or in instances in which the user has waived confidentiality for purposes of third-party payment.

Users have the right to obtain information from their psychological records. However, the records are the property of the psychologist or the facility in which the psychologist works and are, therefore, the responsibility of the psychologist and subject to his or her control.

When the user's intention to waive confidentiality is judged by the professional clinical psychologist to be contrary to the user's best interests or to be in conflict with the user's civil and legal rights, it is the responsibility of the clinical psychologist to discuss the implications of releasing psychological information and to assist the user in limiting disclosure only to information required by the present circumstance.

Raw psychological data (e.g., questionnaire returns or test protocols) in which a user is identified are released only with the written consent of the user or his or her legal representative and released only to a person recognized by the clinical psychologist as qualified and competent to use the data.

Any use made of psychological reports, records, or data for research or training purposes is consistent with this Guideline. Additionally, providers of clinical psychological services comply with statutory confidentiality requirements and those embodied in the American Psychological Association's Ethical Principles of Psychologists (APA, 1981b).

Providers of clinical psychological services remain sensitive to both the benefits and the possible misuse of information regarding individuals that is stored in large computerized data banks. Providers use their influence to ensure that such information is used in a socially responsible manner.

Guideline 3

ACCOUNTABILITY

3.1 The clinical psychologist's professional activity is guided primarily by the principle of promoting human welfare.

INTERPRETATION: Clinical psychologists provide services to users in a manner that is considerate, effective, economical, and humane. Clinical psychologists make their services readily accessible to users in a manner that facilitates the users' freedom of choice.

Clinical psychologists are mindful of their accountability to the sanctioners of clinical psychological services and to the general public, provided that appropriate steps are taken to protect the confidentiality of the service relationships. In the pursuit of their professional activities, they aid in the conservation of human, material, and financial resources.

The clinical psychological service unit does not withhold services to a potential client on the basis of that user's race, color, religion, gender, sexual orientation, age, or national origin. Recognition is given, however, to the following considerations: the professional right

**Exhibit 1–2** continued

of clinical psychologists to limit their practice to a specific category of users (e.g., children, adolescents, women); the right and responsibility of clinical psychologists to withhold an assessment procedure when not validly applicable; and the right and responsibility of clinical psychologists to withhold evaluative, psychotherapeutic, counseling, or other services in specific instances in which their own limitations or client characteristics might impair the effectiveness of the relationship. Clinical psychologists seek to ameliorate through peer review, consultation, or other personal therapeutic procedures those factors that inhibit the provision of services to particular users. When indicated services are not available, clinical psychologists take whatever action is appropriate to inform responsible persons and agencies of the lack of such services.

Clinical psychologists who find that psychological services are being provided in a manner that is discriminatory or exploitative to users and/or contrary to these Guidelines or to state or federal statutes take appropriate corrective action, which may include the refusal to provide services. When conflicts of interest arise, the clinical psychologist is guided in the resolution of differences by the principles set forth in the American Psychological Association's Ethical Principles of Psychologists (APA, 1981b) and "Guidelines for Conditions of Employment of Psychologists" (APA, 1972).

3.2 Clinical psychologists pursue their activities as members of the independent, autonomous profession of psychology.

INTERPRETATION: Clinical psychologists, as members of an independent profession, are responsible both to the public and to their peers through established review mechanisms. Clinical psychologists are aware of the implications of their activities for the profession as a whole. They seek to eliminate discriminatory practices instituted for self-serving purposes that are not in the interest of the users (e.g., arbitrary requirements for referral and supervision by another profession). They are cognizant of their responsibilities for the development of the profession. They participate where possible in the training and career development of students and other providers, participate as appropriate in the training of paraprofessionals or other professionals, and integrate and supervise the implementation of their contributions within the structure established for delivering psychological services. Clinical psychologists facilitate the development of, and participate in, professional standards review mechanisms.

Clinical psychologists seek to work with other professionals in a cooperative manner for the good of the users and the benefit of the general public. Clinical psychologists associated with multidisciplinary settings support the principle that members of each participating profession have equal rights and opportunities to share all privileges and responsibilities of full membership in hospital facilities or other human service facilities and to administer service programs in their respective areas of competence.

3.3 There are periodic, systematic, and effective evaluations of clinical psychological services.

INTERPRETATION: When the clinical psychological service unit is a component of a larger organization, regular evaluation of progress in achieving goals is provided for in the service delivery plan, including consideration of the effectiveness of clinical psychological services relative to costs in terms of use of time and money and the availability of professional and support personnel.

Evaluation of the clinical psychological service delivery system is conducted internally and, when possible, under independent auspices as well. This evaluation includes an assessment of effectiveness (to determine what the service unit accomplished), efficiency (to determine the total costs of providing the services), continuity (to ensure that the services are

*(continues)*

**Exhibit 1–2** continued

appropriately linked to other human services), availability (to determine appropriate levels and distribution of services and personnel), accessibility (to ensure that the services are barrier free to users), and adequacy (to determine whether the services meet the identified needs for such services).

There is a periodic reexamination of review mechanisms to ensure that these attempts at public safeguards are effective and cost efficient and do not place unnecessary encumbrances on the providers or impose unnecessary additional expenses on users or sanctioners for services rendered.

3.4 Clinical psychologists are accountable for all aspects of the services they provide and are responsive to those concerned with these services.

INTERPRETATION: In recognizing their responsibilities to users, and where appropriate and consistent with the users' legal rights and privileged communications, clinical psychologists make available information about, and provide opportunity to participate in, decisions concerning such issues as initiation, termination, continuation, modification, and evaluation of clinical psychological services.

Depending on the settings, accurate and full information is made available to prospective individual or organizational users regarding the qualifications of providers, the nature and extent of services offered, and where appropriate, financial and social costs.

Where appropriate, clinical psychologists inform users of their payment policies and their willingness to assist in obtaining reimbursement. Those who accept reimbursement from a third party are acquainted with the appropriate statutes and regulations and assist their users in understanding procedures for submitting claims and limits on confidentiality of claims information, in accordance with pertinent statutes.

Guideline 4

ENVIRONMENT

4.1 Providers of clinical psychological services promote the development in the service setting of a physical, organizational, and social environment that facilitates optimal human functioning.

INTERPRETATION: Federal, state, and local requirements for safety, health, and sanitation are observed.

As providers of services, clinical psychologists are concerned with the environment of their service unit, especially as it affects the quality of service, but also as it impinges on human functioning when the service unit is included in a larger context. Physical arrangements and organizational policies and procedures are conducive to the human dignity, self-respect, and optimal functioning of users and to the effective delivery of service. Attention is given to the comfort and the privacy of users. The atmosphere in which the clinical psychological services are rendered is appropriate to the service and to the users, whether in an office, clinic, school, industrial organization, or other institutional setting.

**REFERENCES**

American Psychological Association, Committee on Legislation. A model for state legislation affecting the practice of psychology. *American Psychologist,* 1967, *22,* 1095–1103.

American Psychological Association. *Psychology as a profession.* Washington, D.C.: Author, 1968.

**Exhibit 1–2** continued

American Psychological Association, Psychology and national health care. *American Psychologist,* 1971, *26,* 1025–1026.

American Psychological Association. Guidelines for conditions of employment of psychologists. *American Psychologist,* 1972, *27,* 331–334.

American Psychological Association. *Ethical principles in the conduct of research with human participants.* Washington, D.C.: Author, 1973. (a)

American Psychological Association. Guidelines for psychologists conducting growth groups. *American Psychologist,* 1973, *28,* 933. (b)

American Psychological Association. *Standards for educational and psychological tests* Washington, D.C.: Author, 1974. (a)

American Psychological Association. *Standards for providers of psychological services.* Washington, D.C.: Author, 1974. (b)

American Psychological Association. *Education and credentialing in psychology II.* Report of a meeting, June 4-5, 1977. Washington, D.C.: Author, 1977. (a)

American Psychological Association. *Standards for providers of psychological services* (Rev. ed.). Washington, D.C.: Author, 1977. (b)

American Psychological Association. *Criteria for accreditation of doctoral training programs and internships in professional psychology.* Washington, D.C.: Author, 1979 (amended 1980).

American Psychological Association. APA/CHAMPUS *outpatient psychological provider manual* (Rev.ed.). Washington, D.C.: Author, 1981. (a)

American Psychological Association. *Ethical principles of psychologists* (Rev. ed.). Washington, D.C.: Author, 1981. (b)

Conger, J. J. Proceedings of the American Psychological Association, Incorporated, for the year 1975: Minutes of the annual meeting of the Council of Representatives. *American Psychologist,* 1976, *31,* 406–434.

Smith, M.B., & Hobbs, N. *The community and the community mental health center.* Washington, D.C.: American Psychological Association, 1966.



The National Register of Health Service providers in psychology and the National Register of Social Workers have been formed to check on the "fitness" of professionals in their respective professions to practice independently. Some health insurance companies are using the registers as a guide in determining whether or not to reimburse practitioners for services provided to their policy holders.

The diplomate granted by the ABPP, the American Board of Professional Psychology, Inc., is the highest designation of professional competency a psychologist can obtain. The diplomate is granted in four areas of specialization: clinical, counseling, industrial, and organization and school psychology. In order to become a candidate for the diplomate, the psychologist must have completed five years of professional practice after graduating from an APA-approved doctoral program that includes a full-time internship. The candidate must have the endorsement of colleagues attesting to high ethical standards. Once accepted as a candidate, the psychologist must demonstrate expertness in assessment and intervention as well as show an awareness of ethical and professional issues. It is clear that those who are finally awarded diplomate status have demonstrated a high level of competency. Approximately 65 percent of the psychologists who apply for diplomate status ultimately earn their diplomas.

When professionals do not police themselves they invite governmental regulatory agencies to do the job for them. The ultimate purpose is to protect the public from those individuals unqualified to practice.

We have suggested that prior to embarking on independent practice, clinicians pay close attention to the three major domains of attitude, skill, and ethics. These areas have relevance for both public and private practitioners of course, but it is especially important for the independent practitioner to be clear how services are implemented to the public.

In the next section we will focus on how the professional establishes credibility, competency, and communicativeness in the eyes of the public served.

## CREDIBILITY

The first question in the mind of a patient when consulting you is "Can you help me?" The patient must feel confident in your ability to help. It is important that you establish a competency set in the patient's mind. In short, you have to be more than an efficient technician; you have to convey an attitude of a caring professional. Do not fall into the "blank screen" trap in which you want to be a neutral figure so that your patient can project the distortions of personality and interpersonal relations. Such an image is inappropriate for today's independent practitioner. Avoid becoming defensive and threatened, especially during the early sessions when a patient's request for information can be looked upon as a challenge. For example, a patient may ask about your qualifications. The public practitioner is cloaked by the prestige of the institution where the service is delivered and the implicit sanction of the community. The clinician in private practice has neither. At times you may practice in multiple offices and not have your diplomas on display. Patients will inquire about your background. Such questions regarding qualifications can conceal a patient's unsureness about how effective the treatment will be. It is important for you to address the surface questions first. There will be time enough to explore some of the deeper issues when they return. If you brush aside questions regarding your competency and credibility, you may not have the other sessions to get into the deeper material.

Displaying all your diplomas contributes to creating a competency and credibility set in the mind of your client. When the therapy appears at a plateau or the relationship seems stressed, clients often ask about the advisability of consultation. If this occurs, avoid the first impulse to see it as resistance, which it may be, and consider realistic pros and cons of a consultation for your client with another therapist. Consider these pros and cons together with your client. It is wise to be prepared by having a list of colleagues you can call upon for consultation whether initiated by yourself or the patient.

A youngster I was seeing in therapy had among his many symptoms multiple tics. The child's pediatrician and I were both of the opinion that the youngster did not have Tourette's Syndrome. But when his parents raised the issue with me after seeing a television program on the subject, I suggested a consultation with a neurologist who specialized in treating children with this syndrome. The neurologist confirmed the parents' view, put their child on Haldol, with a resulting diminution of many of the tics. The credible practitioner fits the procedure to the patient, not the patient to the procedure.

When presenting your diagnostic formulations to patients or sharing information with them, take a positive stance. For example, let your patients know of your experience in working with clients who have similar problems. This is different from making promises of improvement.

Clinicians who are concerned about giving their patients the wrong impression about their ability to help can create a negative rather than a positive expectancy. We all know about the potent effects of expectancy on the outcome of treatment. Clinicians can make promises to their clients—indeed they must! Do not promise to cure, of course, but making promises, such as the ones below, and keeping them are essential in building up your client's confidence.

- Call back patients when you promise to do so by a certain time or date.
- Follow up when you promise to do so.
- Contact related professionals when you said you would.
- Send out reports on time.

Failing to keep these promises can undermine credibility. Independent practitioners are busy and often do not seem to have enough time in the day. Marking the calendar and appointment book to carry through on these promises is essential as the independent practitioner does not usually have co-workers or secretaries to remind them to perform these tasks.

## COMMUNICATION

Clinicians are acutely aware of the many verbal camouflages such as circumlocution, circumvention, disclaimers, and evasiveness that patients bring with them to the consultation room. However, they often do not pay enough attention to their own style of communication. After an evaluation of their child, a supervisee of mine expressed his findings to the parents in the following way: "I am afraid to have to tell you that your child is suffering from infantile autism." If the "expert" is afraid, how should the parents feel? It is better to tell about problems in a straightforward manner, and in addition, comment on the programs available to help with the problem. For example, "John is a rather immature child who finds it difficult to express his feelings. Such problems are best treated with play therapy." Or "Your headaches are stress related and often a program of stress reduction can significantly affect the frequency and intensity of your headaches. This is what I would suggest . . . "

Be aware of your posture, facial expressions, tone of voice, and hesitancies. All these are, of course, nonverbal behaviors that can convey your feelings and attitudes.

Patients are especially vulnerable to the interfering effects of anxiety during feedback sessions following diagnostic evaluations. Providing the patient with visual aids while discussing your findings is helpful in reducing anxiety and emphasizes the information you are trying to convey. Profile sheets of projective and cognitive tests, figure drawings, feedback checklists, or written reports are some examples. Detailed illustrations of some feedback techniques will be presented in Chapter 6.

## FEEDBACK

Often internists and pediatricians have attempted to assist patients prior to referring them to a mental health specialist. When the patient finally lands in your office, the disability is entrenched or the patient is uncooperative, resistant, or minimizes the need for help. Under these circumstances, do not be afraid to share your impressions with both the patient and the referring physician. This can be a helpful step toward establishing a therapeutic alliance with the patient as well as deflating negative patient feedback to the referral source. Satisfied clients become new referral sources and with the lessening of the stigmata of mental health services, they will refer you to their friends and neighbors should the need arise.

Treat your referral sources with courtesy and concern. Find out their feedback preferences, get back to them quickly, and periodically survey their satisfaction as well as sending them reprints of relevant publications.

Communicating to your patients in a language they can understand and keeping your referral sources abreast of their patients' progress will help label you as a concerned, competent, and credible practitioner.

## SUMMARY

In this chapter we have reviewed some major factors that the independent practitioner should consider prior to entering practice. The clinician has to be equipped with a conceptual schema for understanding the workings of the mind, and conversant with intervention strategies for ameliorating the harmful effects of emotional disabilities. We have also stressed the importance of being aware of your motives and attitudes for entering the marketplace of private practice. Special emphasis was placed on organizational skills as a necessary precursor to good business practices. Finally, we counseled the practitioner to be mindful of the ethical and legal responsibilities that are unique to independent practice. In the chapters that follow, we will zoom in on the specific tactics for putting concepts into practice that will help to establish and maintain a successful private mental health practice.

Chapter 2

# Seven Business Headaches

# 2

The modern-day practitioner has an overabundance of intervention strategies to choose from when tailoring a plan to fit the best interest of his or her client. At times the task may seem overwhelming, yet the competent clinician is by training, temperament, and experience up to the job.

There is less awareness, however, that a similar array of choices is available to the clinician when it comes to making decisions regarding the business aspects of independent practice. Unfortunately, clinicians, by dint of training, temperament, and experience, are not up to making these choices. Because they are unaware of the possibilities that exist, this important aspect of independent practice is often avoided or evaded.

Consider some of the major questions facing a practitioner who decides to devote part or all of his or her professional time to private practice. Where should I situate my office? Would I do better specializing or being a generalist? What type of record system should I have and what is the best way to organize a filing system that takes into consideration present needs and future expansion? How do I determine a fair fee for my services? Is there a best way to bill clients so that I am ensured of payment for my services? What do I do when a client does not pay for my services? What type of equipment will I need?

While the answers to some of these questions may appear simple, for the most part they are complex questions and require ample time and energy on your part in addressing them. Furthermore, experience has taught that these questions have not one simple answer but multiple answers.

Each practitioner decides on the type of practice that will be generated and the amount of time allocated to independent practice. Whether directly or indirectly, the practitioner will be impacted by each of the decisions made to implement his or her professional plans. A good deal of thought is crucial in examining all available alternatives.

Consider, for example, how a menu in a restaurant can acquaint the hungry customer with the many varieties of food available; so, too, a detailed description of any business consideration and realistic resources available to the practitioner can orient him or her to the business issues involved in establishing and maintaining private practice.

## SITUATING YOUR OFFICE

### Where Do You Want To Be?

I asked a successful colleague of mine who maintains a full-time practice of marriage and family counseling how he chose to situate his office in Rochester, New York. Ed, who had received his degree in marriage and family counseling a few years prior to settling in Rochester, decided to become an independent practitioner because he wanted to be his own boss and have greater control over what he did as a clinician. His wife supported him in this decision and together the first thing they considered was the area of the country they wanted to settle in to raise their family. After deciding that they wanted to be in the northeast, they consulted such publications as the *World Almanac, FBI Uniform Crime Reports,* HEW's *Vital Statistics of the U.S.,* and the *Farmer's Almanac,* as well as a number of Chambers of Commerce. They were looking for information on such quality of life indicators as education, medical care, crime, income and wealth, cost of living, recreational facilities, and weather.

This helped them prioritize a few cities. The last step for Ed was to consider realistically whether or not he could make a living practicing marriage and family therapy in any of these communities. Surveying the telephone book provided some information regarding the competition. In addition, he wrote to the United Fund (Community Chest) for a list of agencies they support to gain some ideas about community gate keepers and possible consultations. He also wrote to the directors of clinical training at nearby universities to find out about regional psychological associations. He was then able to contact the organizations' presidents to gain more information about the professional community.

### What Kind of Office Do You Want?

Ed's next step was to decide on an office. He had to consider ease of access and parking facilities. Because his practice was going to "cater" to middle-income families, he was not very concerned about being close to a bus route—he wanted to find an accessible building with ample parking. He traded public transportation for a good location in the suburbs in an office complex that was near an expressway and had its own parking lot. There were two internists and a pediatric group also located in the office complex, and Ed reasoned that these might be possible referral sources.

Ed estimated that it took him about a year to gather the information, decide on a town and move into his professional quarters. These considerations may seem excessive for most practitioners, especially those who are already situated in a community and are considering part-time practice or those who are in transition from public to private practice. Nevertheless, there are some good lessons to be learned. First, know the needs you want satisfied. Second, be aware that change in your professional life affects many other aspects of your life.

An office comes with the job for a public practitioner. More and more clinics, hospitals, and mental health centers permit their employees to conduct independent practice right in their public office as long as it does not conflict with their public duties and responsibilities.

The following is an example of guidelines one agency worked out regarding the use of its facilities by staff for private practice:

> Subject to the demands of work requirements and with written approval of the agency director, full and part time qualified professional employees may conduct a private practice of their profession within the agency. Reimbursement to the agency for space, administrative time and telephone service is to be paid at a rate determined by the agency director. Private practice is not permitted if it conflicts with the employee's work schedule or responsibilities to the agency.

1. Private practice engaged in by any employee of the Mental Health Center must not at any time be in conflict with that person's duties, position or responsibilities as an employee of the agency. It must be conducted outside of regularly scheduled center hours. Each employee engaged in private practice shall submit a time schedule of regularly scheduled center work hours.
2. Any cost accruing to the center for the use of Mental Health Center facilities for private practice shall be promptly reimbursed to the center by the practitioner.
3. Private practitioners while in the employ of the Mental Health Center will be requested to execute a conflict of interest statement. Deviations from the above policies constitute a conflict of interest on the part of the employee and is a basis for dismissal.

Some practitioners prefer to keep their public and private practice completely separate. They provide a clear message that during certain hours the clinician is a private practitioner.

## UTILIZING YOUR OFFICE

The practitioner may prefer to have different furnishings than those found in the "barren institutionalized office" provided by some agencies. Some practitioners see their office and its furnishings as making a definite statement about themselves and their practice. They want to have greater control over this aspect of their practice than they could at the agency in which they practice publicly.

A major consideration in office selection should be cost. If permitted to practice privately in the clinic office, the part-time practitioner usually pays a nominal fee based upon the number of hours the office is used for independent practice.

### Overhead

The figures presented in this section are based on 1983 dollars and can give an idea of what might be expected.

- Office furnishings, maintenance, utilities ($1.30/hr.)
- Receptionists, switchboard ($ .53/hr)
- telephone ($ .10/call)
- telephone listing ($ .68)
- mail (postal rate)
- secretarial ($6.30/hr.)
- copying ($ .05/copy)

Excluding secretarial services, the cost of your public office can be expected to range between 3 and 5 percent of your hourly fee.

The full-time practitioner or clinician who chooses to rent space has to consider that the office rent will probably be the highest monthly overhead cost. While rent will vary according to location—highly populated cities such as New York, Los Angeles, or Chicago have higher costs than such cities as Rochester, Cleveland, or Miami—expect to pay from 10 to 30 percent of your hourly fee. The type of practice you engage in can help determine your space needs. Group therapy will require more space than individual therapy; individual therapy will require more space than outside consultations.

Pressman (1979) has found that a 100 square foot room can comfortably accommodate two chairs, a small desk, and a filing cabinet. This would be sufficient for individual psychotherapy. An office where family therapy would be conducted would require additional space of approximately 50 square feet. One hundred square feet would be sufficient for a waiting room that could accommodate a secretary/receptionist.

The clinician who sees children as well as adults would do well to partition the office so as to provide a play area for the younger clients. Such space need not be large: 4 ft. by 4 ft. would be sufficient.

Some practitioners, especially in large cities, find themselves practicing out of their apartment or using a room in their house. Some possible pitfalls of this arrangement are that it brings too much of your personal life into your practice and a home address on stationery and business cards can convey a lack of professionalism to referral sources. However, remember that Sigmund Freud saw his patients in his house without adverse consequences. A major advantage is financial: namely, the practitioner can deduct from taxes (as an office expense) a portion of his or her living costs. The practitioner not only avoids paying rent but at the same time has the benefit of many of the services of his or her house. If the home office occupies one room in an eight-room house, then 1/8th of the house expenses that relate to the practice, such as heat, telephone, and snow removal, can be deducted as an office expense. The Internal Revenue Service is quite strict about enforcing rules governing the use of one's living quarters for independent practice:

> *#3685 — Business use of home.* Expenses incurred in the use of a taxpayer's home for business purposes are deductible only if they are attributable to the portion of the home used exclusively and regularly as:
>
> 1. The taxpayer's principal place of business, or
> 2. A place of business where the taxpayer meets or deals with customers, clients or patients in the ordinary course of business.
>
> For this purpose, "home" and "place of business" may refer to the taxpayer's actual dwelling or to a nearby separate structure used for business, for example a barn that serves as an artist's studio or a guest house that is utilized as a physician's or an attorney's office.
>
> "Exclusively" means just that: use of the business portion of a home by the taxpayer or members of his or her family for purposes unrelated to business will result in disallowance of business expense deductions (*Federal Tax Guide,* 1983).

Most mental health practitioners do not make rounds or house calls, and driving from home to the office is not tax deductible. However, should you drive from your house to your public office, back to your private office, then to your public office in the same day, travel expenses between offices can be deducted.

The beginning part-time private practitioner who uses an agency office certainly has the advantage of paying reasonable rent, and in many instances has available the use of much furniture and equipment that would otherwise have to be purchased. If you are able to keep the public and private aspects of your practice separate and clear of interest conflicts, the advantages of using your public office become even greater. You have the opportunity of scheduling appointments at the beginning and end of your day and during noon. If you extend your day, you can have dinner in the cafeteria and continue to see your private patients later in the evening.

An informal survey among practitioners in the Rochester, New York area (an area which is frequently used to pretest new products) suggests that the independent practitioner generally starts out on a part-time basis and situates his or her practice in the clinic or hospital office that the institution provides.

Space sharing is a variant of this approach. Some clinicians rent office space from colleagues who find that their existing office space is more than they need or that they are away from the office a number of hours a week. The part-time clinician can thus significantly lower monthly overhead and find office quarters that are more pleasant than the facilities available at his or her agency. Furthermore, this arrangement can provide the beginning practitioner with a furnished office, thus minimizing such initial costs as chairs, desk, etc. Secretarial help, such as a typist or receptionist, is also often available. An established practitioner is usually willing to be of assistance to a newcomer, especially if the beginning practitioner's services complement the office's existing ones, such as a psychiatrist renting space to a social worker or clinical psychologist, both of whom can provide complementary clinical services (psychological testing and case work).

## STRUCTURING YOUR BUSINESS PRACTICE

Recent surveys have clearly demonstrated that more and more practitioners are considering entering independent practice. Boneau and Cuca (1974) reported that 13% percent of APA members surveyed considered themselves as principally private practitioners. Surveys conducted only three years later showed a tripling of APA members who said they were engaged in private practice. Gottfredson and Dyer (1978) reported that 20 percent of the psychologists surveyed in 1978 indicated they engaged in independent practice and Wellner and Mills (1977) found that 25 percent of surveyed psychologists reported that they engaged in independent practice.

In considering the type of business structure to be established, it is wise to remember that lawyers and accountants are helpful consultants to the practicing clinician. Expert practitioners know how valuable it is for their clients to anticipate possible problems and/or traumatic occurrences. The same reasoning holds true when considering business practices. Before putting your name on the dotted line, consult with an attorney. Before setting up systems that will impact on tax returns, consult an accountant. A dearly beloved attorney friend of mine advised that I take the same advice that I give to my clients, namely to be proactive rather than reactive to problems.

There are basically three major business structures for the practitioner to consider: corporative, partnership, or solo.

### Corporation

In order to incorporate, you are required to file papers of incorporation according to state rules and regulations. While each state has different laws governing incorporating, it is now possible for professionals to become incorporated as either professional corporations (PC) or professional associations (PA). There is usually considerable expense both in terms of legal fees and corporate fees. Some legal fees can run into thousands of dollars. A corporation's major advantage of limited liability (owners of a corporation are not liable for the corporation's debts) is far outweighed by the cost. The major gain the professional has for incorporating is tax sheltering and pension plans. However, if the corporation does not show a large income, there is basically little money to pay for such benefits and, furthermore, any profits over expenses that the corporation shows are taxed. Thus, in effect, the professional pays a dual income tax. Most practitioners, especially those in part-time practice, have not incorporated. They consider forming either a solo practice or a partnership.

### Partnership

Two or more practitioners who are interested in working together can verbally (but more often than not in writing) form a partnership. The partnership is basically an agreed-upon plan for sharing income and expenses. The partnership will provide income to each of its members, who will be taxed separately and also will be liable for the debts of the partnership. There are variations of partnerships, so that it is possible for partners to form a partnership without assuming complete liability of the partnership. Often psychologists agree to form what are known as "loose partnerships" whereby each member is basically a solo practitioner but agrees to share expenses. They maintain separate records, bill their clients independently, and cultivate their own referral sources.

### Solo Practice

Solo practitioners are not governed by state or local rules. All that usually is required is a license or certificate to go into business. Of course, the solo practitioner assumes all liabilities and responsibilities for the practice and by the same token reaps all of the rewards. As we noted in Chapter 1, solo practitioners who plan to spend full time in practice have to be careful not to become isolated lone wolves. They must budget some time for contacts with other psychologists or mental health professionals. They cannot afford to miss the new ideas and stimulation from the give-and-take public practitioners. Part-time practitioners do not run that risk—opportunities for stimulation, consultation, supervision, and in-service training are available as part of their day-to-day public responsibilities.

## OWNING OR RENTING

Just as a family looking for a place to live has to decide whether to rent or purchase, so does the practitioner when considering an office. Renting an office unburdens you of many of the responsibilities for repairs. Furthermore, you need not worry when on vacation that something may go wrong with the office building you own.

Most renters are required to sign a lease, which should include a description of:

- the property rented
- dates specifying beginning and termination of the lease
- specific responsibilities of each party for such things as repairs, replacement, and alterations
- whether or not the property comes with utilities and equipment furnished by the landlord
- amount of rent to be paid
- whether or not the tenant can make renovations or alter the decor
- a statement about breaking the lease and whether or not the premises could be sublet

Give some thought to the future. While the young practitioner may be renting more space than needed and initially overpaying, remember that office expense does not increase as the volume of your business increases. Rather it becomes less costly as an expense against income. Effective practices spend from 5 to 8 percent of their gross income for office rent. New practitioners find their end cost higher, whereas those who have been practicing for a longer period of time find it somewhat lower. As with most legal documents—and the lease is a legal document—it is wise to have it carefully examined by your attorney. It is also best for a new practitioner not to enter into a long-term lease. Beware of the lease that has escalation clauses requiring cost of living increases in rent. It is also to your advantage to see that escape clauses are available.

Most mental health practitioners are not in the position to construct or purchase an office building for use as their full-time clinical practice. The major advantage of building or buying centers around the investment in property and has little relationship to the clinical practice. It is an investment in property with your capital, hopefully appreciating over time while providing the tax benefits from depreciation. Expenses involved in repairing, refurnishing, and upkeeping your property can be applied to the cost of running your business. Remember that ownership may restrict moving elsewhere. For example, if your space has become too small, or the area changes, or you decide to become involved in a different practice with other clientele, or an interesting offer comes along from the public sector, your move will be more difficult.

## FURNISHINGS

The wise practitioner gives almost as much thought to the office furnishings as to its location. This is essential for two reasons: first, because profit or income is the net result or difference between expenses (overhead) and billings, and second, because the way you package your services, which includes more than the personal involvement with your clients and patients, is extremely important.

The furniture and office environment convey a message about you to the clients served. For example, while in the waiting room the client may be anxious, worried, and unsure about his or her first introduction to you. A properly furnished waiting area may help to tone down some of the discomforts. Similarly, if children are your primary clients, a neat and overly tidy "childproof" office may be uninviting and inhibiting.

In addition, your office is your home away from home and thus it is important for you to give consideration to your own comfort. The area in which you do your professional work, your reading and writing, should be pleasant and comfortable.

The part-time practitioner who is considering venturing into full-time practice or leaving the quarters provided by the employing institution can be especially vulnerable if the many office expenses are not realized. The items discussed in the following sections are those that independent practitioners should consider.

## Furniture

### *Desks*

Desks come in various sizes and types. Some practitioners prefer large executive conference type desks, which are generally 6 ft. by 3 ft., whereas others prefer smaller desks that can accommodate a patient seated at the side to facilitate psychological testing. Some practitioners who do a good deal of marital and family counseling have foregone a desk for a credenza and circular table. If you go the route of secretary/typist/receptionist, then an additional desk will be required. This is usually a special desk with a typewriter compartment.

The cost of a desk can vary greatly depending upon its size, whether it is purchased from the Salvation Army or similar sources, personally refinished, or part of a designer's package. However, an attractive, functional, executive desk can usually be purchased for a few hundred dollars.

### *Chairs*

The chairs you use both for yourself and your patients should be comfortable, durable, and if possible, attractive. In addition to your chair, one or two deep comfortable chairs and one or two relatively firm hard-backed seats will be sufficient. The price range can vary from $10.00 for metal folding or stackable chairs to hundreds of dollars for plush upholstered chairs.

### *Storage Units*

Today, filing cabinets and bookcases come in an assortment of sizes and colors. Large stationery stores, office supply outlets, department stores, and catalogue houses provide you with a wealth of information on prices, styles, and availability.

## Telephone Answering Service

It is a good bet that when the phone rings most mental health practitioners are busy with a client or away from the office. If you engage a secretary or have an arrangment for this service at your public office, then there usually is no problem. However, if you are like most practitioners, especially those not in full-time practice, the question becomes "answering service or answering machine?" The services are personal, they can question the caller for pertinent information, and they can contact you rapidly in an emergency. Medical colleagues can be helpful in steering you to a reliable and ethical answering service. The major drawback to choosing an answering service is the cost when compared with an answering machine. Answering machines range from below $100.00 to over $500.00 depending upon the make and features. Some machines can be activated from a distant phone and will play back your messages, while other machines will permit you to change the message through remote control. A major disadvantage of this system is that many people dislike talking to "electronic robots."

The recorded message you leave becomes extremely important. The message should be in your own voice, short, and mention when you will return and where you can be reached in an emergency. The following is one possible example: "Hello, you have reached the offices of Dr. Kissel. I am away from the office and will be returning this afternoon/evening/morning. If you leave your name and phone number at the beep, I will return your call promptly. If this is an emergency, I can be reached at (telephone number). Thank you."

**Paper Supplies**

Stationery, business cards, announcements, and billing forms will be discussed at length in the section on record keeping and marketing. They are mentioned now to remind the practitioner that these expenses have to be considered. Although they are not major ones, they are still important.

Folders and notepapers are also relatively inexpensive items that can make your life a little easier if given some forethought. A system using plain manila folders into which you throw papers and notes tends to become messy, with the likelihood of important information being lost. Folders that have fasteners are more acceptable. It is a simple procedure to hole-punch tablets that can be inserted into the file. Pencils, pens, appointment calendars, index cards, and index card files are some other stationery costs.

**Recording**

The cost of a telephone, its installation and monthly charges, is a necessary expense.

Although helpful for dictating your reports and recording interviews, dictating equipment such as a tape recorder or dictaphone is not a necessity.

A good typewriter, if you engage a secretary or do your own typing, is another item that has to be considered. Serviceable electric typewriters can be purchased for a few hundred dollars but it is your reports, what they say, and *how they look,* that are important. Poorly typed and disorganized reports can lead the reader to question your professionalism. Good office machines start at considerably higher prices but in the long run are worth the added expense.

## CHOOSING SPECIAL PROFESSIONAL MATERIALS

### Play Therapy

Contrary to popular opinion, you do not need an elaborate playroom or a toy chest of expensive items to work with children. My first office had an alcove with sufficient room for a table, two chairs, a cabinet with a door, and some open shelving. It is important to have at least one storage area that is closed, because open closets filled with play materials are distracting and can interfere with diagnostic evaluations. Playroom articles such as blackboard, bulletin board, and sink are helpful. They are desirable but not necessary. An area as small as 4 ft. x 4 ft. is sufficient, especially if it opens into your larger office. Of course, a room 8 ft. by 10 ft. with running water would be even more desirable.

Exhibit 2–1 provides a list of materials commonly found in playrooms. The list is arranged according to a "diagnostic" schema that will help the therapist select a play item.

**Exhibit 2–1** Play Materials

| *Loosening* | *Modeling* | *Tightening Up* |
|---|---|---|
| Clay/Play Dough | Puppets | Construction |
| Crayons | Animal | Leather |
| Paints | People | Sewing |
| Paper | Dollhouse | Models |
| Finger-Paints | Furniture | Glue |
| Blocks | People | Cards |
| Darts, Dart Board | Doctor Kit | Board Games |
| Punching Bag | Play Money | "Sorry" |
| Water | Blackboard | Checkers |
| Sandbox | | Any Game with Rules |
| | | Mirrors |
| | | Audio-Visual Tape Recorder |
| | | Balls |

Loosening up items are helpful in stimulating children who are overly anxious, depressed, or inhibited. Items that provide structure, direction, and rules are helpful in introducing control into meetings with children who are overactive, distractible, and action oriented.

## Biofeedback

Considerably more nonmedically as well as medically trained mental health specialists are appreciating the value of behaviorally oriented biofeedback in the treatment of a number of stress-related problems, such as headaches, weight loss, and pain. Although many advertisers have suggested that biofeedback equipment is so simple to use that "they can be bought for home use or for your secretary to use with patients," this is not accurate. For the most part the opposite is true. The application of biofeedback without proper training in physiology, learning theory, interviewing techniques, and indications and contraindications for the use of biofeedback is nonprofessional and can be harmful. Fortunately, the majority of clinicians who use biofeedback are trained and have had much experience with instrumentation, usually under supervision and within the confines of a university.

There are some major costs, apart from training, which the practitioner needs to consider. The Autogenic Corporation, 809 Allston Way, Berkeley, California, 94710, offers a number of models that are able to generate electromyogram (EMG) and temperature readings. Audio and visual output are provided in packages starting at about $1,000.00. In addition, a reclining couch or chair, and an ottoman are also required and they can be purchased for $100.00 to $300.00. For under $2,000 a clinician can comfortably outfit an office with biofeedback equipment.

Thought Technology, 2193 Clifton Avenue, Suite 131, Montreal, Quebec, Canada, H4A2N5, has introduced a very serviceable, hand-held, battery-operated monitor. It comes with a thermostat for measuring temperature, a readout meter, and electrodes. This miniature portable apparatus measures galvanic skin resistance (GSR) and temperature, providing both audio and visual feedback, and it can be used in the office or loaned to the patient for practice at home. This apparatus is fairly inexpensive, costing under $100.00.

Even though clinicians often invest more for biofeedback equipment than other equipment, there has been a profound interest and great acceptance of the behaviorally oriented biofeedback techniques for the management of many stress-related problems.

## Psychological Testing

Although some practitioners confine their independent practice exclusively to psychotherapy, the majority of private practitioners, especially psychologists, devote at least part of their time to psychological testing. While psychologists know the type of assessment techniques they will use to answer a specific referral question, they are less familiar with who publishes the tests and where they may be purchased. The costs of items to be described below are based on current catalog prices and, of course, can be expected to change.

### *Intelligence Tests*

• *The Wechsler Intelligence Scales*—The Wechsler Adult Intelligence Scale-R, Wechsler Intelligence Scale for Children-R, and the Wechsler Pre-School and Primary Scale of Intelligence are the most used psychological tests. They can be purchased by qualified psychologists from the Psychological Corporation, 757 Third Avenue, New York, New York 10017. The costs of the materials are:

| | |
|---|---|
| WAIS-R Kit | $55.00 |
| Additional forms, 100 | 10.25 |
| WISC-R Kit | 69.00 |
| Additional forms, 100 | 20.50 |
| WPPSI Kit | 60.00 |
| Additional forms, 100 | 20.50 |

• *The Stanford-Binet Intelligence Scale*—Form L-M, although not used as widely, nevertheless is a major individually administered test. It can be ordered from Houghton Mifflin Co., One Beacon Street, Boston, Massachusetts 02107. The cost is:

| | |
|---|---|
| Stanford Binet Scale | $99.00 |
| Additional forms, 35 | 6.25 |

• *The Slossen Intelligence Test*—This individually administered test consisting of 194 items, presented in an ascending order of difficulty, was designed to provide a quick estimate of general intelligence. The test takes approximately 20 minutes to administer and score. It can be obtained from Slossen Educational Publications, 140 Pine Street, East Aurora, New York 14052. The cost is:

| | |
|---|---|
| SIT Kit | $13.50 |
| Additional forms, 20 | 2.50 |

• *The Peabody Picture Vocabulary Test*—The PPVT was designed to test for general intelligence when a limited amount of time was available. It does not require the examinee to respond verbally. The test is available from American Guidance Services, Inc., Publisher's Building, Circle Pines, Minnesota, 55404. The cost is:

| | |
|---|---|
| PPVT Kit | $22.00 |
| Additional forms, 50 | 4.25 |

• *Raven Progressive Matricies*—This test is presented as a relatively culture-free test of general intelligence and can be administered either individually or in a group. It takes approximately 45 minutes to an hour to administer and score, and can be purchased from the Psychological Corporation. The cost is:

| | |
|---|---|
| RPM Kit (specimen set) | $ 9.00 |
| Additional forms, 10 | 30.75 |

*Personality Tests*

• *Rorschach*—The Rorschach Ink Blot Test is the most widely used and most eminent projective technique available to assess personality development, integration, and level of emotional disturbance. The set of ten ink blot cards and location charts can be purchased from Grune and Stratton, Inc., 381 Park Avenue South, New York, New York 10016. The cost is:

| | |
|---|---|
| Rorschach Kit | $28.50 |
| Additional forms, location charts, 100 | 11.00 |

• *Thematic Apperception Test*—This projective personality assessment tool has one version for adults (TAT) and one for children (CAT). The stories examinees create to go with the standard pictures reveal important information about their needs, value systems, and especially attitudes toward significant figures and situations in the environment. The test consists of a set of pictures, 31 in the TAT version and 10 in the CAT version, and can be ordered from the Psychological Corporation. The costs are:

| | |
|---|---|
| TAT Kit | $12.50 |
| Additional forms | none |
| CAT Kit | 49.00 |
| Additional forms, 25 | 5.25 |

• *Sentence Completion Test*—This semiprojective, semiobjective personality test has many versions. The Rotter Incomplete Sentence Blank, which has a high school, college, and adult version, can be objectively scored along three dimensions: conflict or unhealthy response, neutral response, and positive or healthy response. Like most sentence completion tests it takes less than 30 minutes to complete. This test can be obtained from the Psychological Corporation. The cost is:

| | |
|---|---|
| ISB Kit | $ 4.50 |
| Additional forms, 100 | 10.00 |

• *Minnesota Multiphasic Personality Inventory*—This most widely used objective personality test can be group or individually administered, hand or machine scored, and interpreted by a clinician or a computer. A number of abbreviated and short forms have been generated from the original 550-item version. The basic test can be obtained from the Psychological Corporation. The cost is:

| | |
|---|---|
| MMPI Kit (specimen set) | $7.00 |
| Additional forms (inventory books, 1) | 4.50 |
| (answer sheets, 50) | 7.00 |

A number of publishers, including the Psychological Corporation, have their own systems for computerized scoring and interpretation that require specialized answer sheets. Samples for a nominal fee are available from:

(1) Caldwell Reports
3122 Santa Monica Blvd.
Santa Monica, California 90404
(2) WPS Test Reports
1231 Wilshire Blvd.
Los Angeles, California 90025
(3) NCS Interpretive Scoring Systems
P.O. Box 1416
Minneapolis, Minnesota 55440

• *16-P-F Test*—This is another widely used objective personality inventory that provides the clinician with information about normal as well as abnormal personality functioning. Questions are hand or mechanically scored.

Computerized interpretations and reports are available. The test can be obtained from Institute for Personality and Ability Testing, 1602 Coronado Drive, Champaign, Illinois 61820. The cost is:

| | |
|---|---|
| Testing Kit (specimen set) | 9.00 |
| Additional forms (test booklets, 25) | 13.50 |
| (answer sheets, 50) | 4.90 |

*Graphomotor Tests*

• *Bender Visual Motor Gestalt Test*—The nine designs that have to be copied on an 8½ by 11 inch blank piece of paper were originally developed as a test for "organicity" but have since come to have multiple uses. The set of cards and interpretive manual can be obtained from the American Orthopsychiatric Association, 735 Broadway, New York, New York. The cost is:

| | |
|---|---|
| Bender-Gestalt Kit | $17.00 |

A number of detailed and norm-based scoring systems are available to help with interpretation. A developmental scoring system, developed and normed by Elizabeth Koppitz, is a feature of *The Bender-Gestalt Test for Young Children,* published by Grune and Stratton. G.R. Pascal and B. Suttel have published a similar objectified approach to scoring the test when the examinee is an adult. Their version is available from the Psychological Corporation.

• *Human Drawing Test*—A blank sheet of 8½ by 11 inch paper and a pencil are the equipment necessary to administer this test. Instructions to examinees can vary from requesting them to "draw a picture of a person" to having them "make a picture of themselves and every member in their family doing something." A number of manuals can be helpful to the clinician in interpreting the graphomotor production:

- Goodenough, F. *Measurement of Intelligence.* New York: World Book, 1926.
- Harris, D.B. *Children's Drawings as Measures of Intellectual Maturity.* New York: Harcourt, Brace, 1963.
- Mackover, K. *Personality Projection in the Drawings of the Human Figure.* Springfield, Ill.: Charles C Thomas, 1949.
- Burns, R.C., and Kaufman, S.H. *Actions, Styles and Symbols in Kinetic Family Drawings* (K-F-D). New York: Brunner/Mazel.

*Vocational Tests*

• *Strong-Campbell Interest Inventory*—This is a revision of the first of the vocational interest blanks to be developed and many clinicians believe it to be the most valid. Four hundred occupationally related items are presented and the examinee has to indicate if he or she agrees, disagrees, or is indifferent to each item. Although it can be hand scored, the Strong is extremely time consuming to score, as each item has to be scored for each available occupational key. Machine scoring, although costly, is more practical. The test is available from NCS Interpretive Scoring Systems, P.O. Box 1416, Minneapolis, Minnesota 55440. The costs are:

| | |
|---|---|
| Strong Kit (reusable booklets, 50) | $16.50 |
| Additional forms (answer sheets, 50) | 13.00 |
| (manual) | 8.25 |
| Scoring Cost (profile report) | 4.00 |
| (interpretive report) | 10.00 |

• *Kuder Preference Record Form*—This test uses a forced-choice approach that requires the examinee to choose which of a series of alternative activities is liked least and most. Examinees can score the test themselves, which can facilitate interpretation. The Kuder is available from SRA, Inc., 259 East Erie Street, Chicago, Illinois 60611. The cost is:

| | |
|---|---|
| Kuder Kit (specimen set) | $ 5.00 |
| Additional Forms (includes scoring 20) | 51.80 |

*Achievement Tests*

• *Wide Range Achievement Test*—This is a favorite of clinical and school psychologists as it takes a minimum amount of educational expertise to administer and score. The WRAT tests for ability in reading, arithmetic, and spelling and is normed by age, not grade level. It is also relatively short, taking approximately 15 to 20 minutes to administer. The test is available from Jastak Associates, Inc., 1526 Gilpin Avenue, Wilmington, Delaware 19806. The cost is:

| | |
|---|---|
| WRAT Kit | $16.00 |
| Additional forms, 50 | 6.90 |

• *Key Math Diagnostic Arithmetic Test*—This is an individually administered mathematics test that provides the examiner with information on achievement level and mathematical process. It is particularly helpful in designing remedial programs for students with mathematical deficiencies. The test is obtained from American Guidance Services, Inc. The cost is:

| | |
|---|---|
| Key Math Kit | $31.00 |
| Additional forms, 25 | 2.90 |

• *Standard Reading Inventory*—This test requires that the administrator have knowledge of the reading process. It provides specific standards for obtaining frustration, instructional, and independent reading levels. It is extremely helpful in designing remedial reading programs as it provides information on vocabulary, comprehension, speed, and oral and silent reading levels. The test is available from Klamath Printing Company, Klamath Falls, Oregon 97604. The cost is:

| | |
|---|---|
| SRI Kit | $7.00 |
| Additional forms, 20 | 7.00 |

*Specific Learning Disability Tests*

Although there is no one single test that diagnoses a specific learning disability, a few tests have been widely used by psychologists to help them formulate a diagnosis of learning disability and make suggestions to school personnel for remediation.

• *Illinois Test of Psycholinguistic Abilities*— This individually administered test is about as lengthy and complex as any of the nine primary and two additional subtests that cover a number of key language abilities theoretically related to the reading process. The key areas are reception, association, and expression. These areas are tested in the auditory, visual, verbal, and nonverbal modes. Automatic processes such as memory, closure, and sound blending are also tested. The ITPA is available from the University of Illinois Press, Urbana, Illinois 61801. The cost is:

| | |
|---|---|
| ITPA Kit | $120.00 |
| Additional forms, 25 | 12.00 |

• *Frostig Developmental Test of Visual Perception*—Based on the developmental theories of Hans Werner and Jean Piaget, this test focuses on the perceptual processes related to reading. It can be group or individually administered to children between the ages of 2½ and 10; it provides scores that are norm based in five areas of visual perception: eye-hand coordination, figure ground, constancy of shape, position in space, and spatial relations.

The test can be purchased from Consulting Psychologists Press, 557 College Avenue, Palo Alto, California 94306.

| | |
|---|---|
| Frostig Kit (specimen set) | $ 6.00 |
| Additional forms, 25 | 10.00 |
| 100 | 38.50 |

## ACCOUNTS RECEIVABLE

The private practitioner must come to grips with the practical and emotional problems of the money question: how much to charge for services, how to bill clients, what to do when they do not promptly pay for services, and what to do when they do not pay for services at all. While there are no ironclad rules, there are some helpful guidelines. In this section we will consider fee setting, billing, and collection.

### Fee Setting

The first thing the practitioner needs to do is recognize his or her own attitude toward the relationship between money and his work as a practicing professional. Sigmund Freud, one of the earliest private mental health practitioners, gave the following advice to analysts:

> The analyst does not dispute that money is to be regarded first and foremost as the means by which life is supported and power is obtained, but he maintains that besides this, powerful sexual factors are involved in the values set upon it; he may expect, therefore, that money questions will be treated by cultured people in the same manner as sexual matters—with the same inconsistency, prudishness and hypocrisy. He is therefore determined beforehand not to concur in this attitude and in his dealings with patients to treat of money matters with the same matter of course frankness that he wishes to induce in them towards matters relating to sexual life. By voluntarily introducing the subject of fees and stating the price for which he gives his time, he shows the patient that he himself has cast aside false shame in these matters. Ordinary prudence then demands that the sums to be paid should not be allowed to accumulate until they are very large, but that payment should be made at fairly short regular intervals (a month or so). It is well known that the value of treatment is not enhanced in the patient's eyes if a very low fee is asked. (1953, pp. 351–352)

The practitioner can benefit from a number of sources of information in attempting to arrive at a reasonable fee for service. The recent survey (Psychotherapy Finances, 1978) of over 1,000 mental health practitioners, of which 80 percent were either psychologists or social workers and the remaining 20 percent marriage counselors, psychiatrists, and pastoral counselors, revealed that fees in general are slightly higher in the south and west and lower in the east and midwest. The minimum figure per hour for psychiatrists was $55.00, for psychologists $45.00, and for social workers $35.00. Some professionals prefer to charge fees similar to their colleagues and periodically poll them to consider the community's standard. The part-time private practitioner working at a mental health agency has ready access to professionals of other disciplines and can gear a fee schedule that is comparable to what other professionals charge for similar services.

Psychiatrists tend to have the highest fees, followed by psychologists, social workers, marriage therapists, and guidance counselors. A nonmedical mental health practitioner, however, need not set fees below that of the medically oriented practitioner but can successfully increase his or her fees depending on education, subspecialty, and expertise. For example, a clinical psychologist who has earned a diplomate (American Board of Professional Psychologists, Inc.) can command a fee on the par of physician colleagues. Another source of information is health insurance plans, such as Blue Shield, Travelers, or Aetna, which have schedules of maximum reimbursable rates for psychotherapy, consultation, and diagnostic workups. In some states insurance companies will not reimburse patients for mental health services unless the services were rendered by a physician or under the supervision of a physician. It is incidental whether or not the physician was trained in diagnosing and treating mental illness or emotional disturbance. This practice has begun to change. At both the state and federal level, fee for service by psychologists has gained statutory recognition. Twenty-nine states plus the District of Columbia have passed Freedom of Choice laws as of 1983 requiring third-party payees (insurance companies) to reimburse psychologists for their services.

Public Law 93-112 recognizes the "physician or licensed psychologist" as qualified to provide assessment and/or restorative services. The regulation implementing PL 93-112, the Health Maintenance Organization Act of 1973, lists clinical psychologists as recognized practitioners.

The recent changes in federal and state laws have also provided the nonmedical private mental health practitioner the option of assignment of fees. By agreeing to bill at the rate set by the insurance company, the practitioner gets reimbursed directly by the insurance carrier. The benefits to the practitioner include assurance of payment, minimal discussion with the patient about fees, and the avoidance of costly and at times unpleasant collection procedures. The disadvantage is that fees are usually considerably lower than the fee the practitioner might charge. If your patient has this type of third-party coverage, you do not have to agree to assignment, or charge fees lower than you would normally charge for such services. You have to make clear that the patient is responsible for paying the difference between the normal fee and the one that the carrier provides. The contract for service is between the practitioner and the patient. Thus, the ultimate responsibility for the payment of professional services rests with the patient and not with the insurance company.

A special consideration needs to be given to charging clients for psychodiagnostic work. Considerable time and effort are spent "invisible to the patient" in scoring, interpreting, integrating, and reporting on the findings. This can take as much time as the administration of the test to the client. In general, a typical battery takes approximately four hours. My standard clinical battery consists of intelligence tests, (WISC-R, WAIS-R, or WPPSI), two projective tests (one of which is the Rorschach), a clinical or play interview, and visual motor techniques (Bender-Gestalt, Graham-Kendall).

Whatever your fees, a schedule of fees must be available to the consumer upon demand. Have your fees typed and posted with your receptionist or if, as many independent practitioners, you do not have a receptionist, your schedule still should be typed and readily available. The schedule should list the charges for each service offered. Table 2–1 provides an example of a fee schedule.

**Table 2–1** Fee Schedule*

| *Description* | *Fee* |
|---|---|
| Psychotherapy, individual session, 1 hour | $ 55.00 |
| Psychotherapy, individual session, each additional half-hour | 25.00 |
| Psychotherapy, group session, per psychotherapy session, 1½ to 2 hours | 25.00 |
| Family session, 1½ hours | 75.00 |
| Psychological evaluation (including testing, interpretation, and report) | 275.00 |
| Consultation and report | 75.00 |

*Based on 1983 dollars

Many private practitioners worry about creating the impression that they are overly concerned about money and less about the well-being of their client. They do not want the financial aspect to infringe upon the clinical aspects of their practice. In reality, especially for the independent practitioner, both are interrelated. Some practitioners find it difficult to realistically appraise the work of their service; others may question whether or not they are worth the amount of money being charged by some colleagues; yet others feel threatened by questions concerning the "high cost of service." Many referrals come from child care workers, such as pediatricians, who are unaccustomed to the cost of mental health services. They are more familiar with the seemingly low cost of pediatric care.

It is helpful to discuss the cost of service with each family, describing the units of service, the time frame, and how much the service will cost. I do this at the end of the initial interview. I also instruct my receptionist to be frank and open with clients who ask about fees when making an initial appointment, rather than deferring the answers. Most people who consult a mental health expert are upset and having problems. I find it inappropriate to immediately discuss the fee with them. After talking for a period of time, yet before they become overly committed or involved, it is important for them to know the cost of service.

The question of failed and canceled appointments can be introduced at the same time a contract for service is made with the client. While practice varies, most practitioners bill for failed appointments but not for cancellations. I do not charge for canceled appointments so long as the client cancels prior to our agreed-upon time. Reasons are not required but they are often volunteered. Initially I required patients to call within 24 hours and got many excuses when they called just prior to their time.

Patients who repeatedly cancel are not interested in therapy or are not able to use it profitably. They would be better served by you confronting them with their behavior, even though you risk their decision to terminate service. However, those patients who have failed to contact me have paid for their failed appointments, and it has not ended our relationship.

Fees are not static—overtime practitioners can be expected to raise their fees. Generally, it is unwise to raise the normal fees of an existing client. The contract for service is "in force" until termination, and an increase in the client's fees during service can be expected to be met with resentment and anger.

## Billing

Billing can be an extremely complex or a very simple procedure, depending upon the size of the practice. Whatever the amount of income of the practice, the billing system has to minimize errors and maximize control. Essentially, all billing systems, whether simple, elaborate, or computerized, require that the practitioner keep a record of daily appointments indicating who was seen, post the fee charged or paid to the patient's account, and then communicate to the patient the amount for such service. The major question most practitioners have is how to use a minimum amount of time and energy on billing without losing accuracy.

While community agencies and large group practices, where billing runs into hundreds of thousands of dollars, have found posting machines and computerized billing an efficient approach, most independent practitioners generate considerably less income and find such elaborate procedures unnecessary. Although it is a luxury for the part-time practitioner and unnecessary for the full-time practitioner whose billing is under $50,000, it is possible to purchase commercial, preprinted receipt ledger systems for $100–$200.

The following system is both economical and accurate. The first component involves an appointment calendar such as a weekly reminder, where daily appointments can be listed. The second component is a monthly log sheet that provides a space for the patient's name, the date of service, the cost of service, and whether it is to be billed or paid. The final component consists of a loose-leaf binder where each patient's account is kept. Monthly entries are made to each patient's account sheet from the log sheet. They provide the basis for sending out bills to patients who do not pay after each visit, and also afford sufficient control over accounts to prevent serious collection problems from occurring. Each patient's account sheet should have the name of the patient, address of the patient, phone number, and diagnosis. The latter is important especially when third-party payees want a summary of business activity and relevant clinical information such as diagnosis, type of visit, and length of visit.

Whenever your patient pays immediately following a visit it saves billing costs, provides you with immediate funds, and, most important, avoids the risk of bad debts. However, not all practitioners or patients are comfortable with such a procedure. Although it is more traditional to bill patients monthly, I find that by matter-of-factly offering patients the choice between monthly billing and pay-as-you-go, more and more patients are choosing to pay visit by visit. I also prefer to personally hand clients their bill rather than have it mailed or presented by the receptionist. I have found this procedure convenient for the following reasons: it introduces reality, makes it easier to focus on delinquent accounts, makes it easier for clients to inquire directly about money matters, and minimizes postage expenses.

## Collections

Regardless of how promptly and effectively you collect for your services, whether by billing or immediately after your service is rendered, some of your patients, usually a small percentage, will not pay bills promptly. An even smaller percentage of your delinquent patients will refuse to pay their bills and require collection agencies or litigation. Some approaches practitioners have used with delinquent accounts are:

- stickers attached to their bills
- collection form letters
- lawyers' letters
- collection agencies
- attorneys
- Small Claims Court

Before considering the more costly approaches involving collection agents, lawyers, or Small Claims Court, let us examine some successful ways of avoiding patient animosity, and avoiding having to share your fee with a collector.

It is especially important when attempting to collect your late fee to allow your patient to save face by minimizing shame and permitting him or her to maintain dignity. It is equally important to maintain your professional image. The slow-paying patient often has the attitude, "Why bother to pay my doctor's bill this month when I can pay it next month?" The finance company would be paid or it would repossess the car; a department store would penalize the late payer with interest charges; the independent practitioner patiently waits. A successful procedure is to bill the client for two consecutive months, and if no payment is received after the second month (approximately 60 days after the service), attach a brief note with the bill. If there is no response to this note within two weeks, send a letter. Phone if there is no response to the second letter. If the telephone call doesn't bring results, the next step would be a collection agency, lawyer, or Small Claims Court. Remember, persistence and a structured approach plus some of your time is still less costly than a collection agency.

The following is an example of a billing note after two months: "Your balance of $250.00 is past due. If you have a question regarding this, please call the office." If this brief note does not meet with success, then a more forceful letter can be sent. An example of such a letter would be: "Your past due balance of $250.00 is now delinquent. Would you please pay your bill or call the office by [give a date no longer than two weeks from the date your letter is mailed] to discuss the matter."

Now let us consider the telephone call. Begin by asking the patient how he or she is doing, and then make the statement that you have been reviewing your accounts and have noticed that the patient has not paid his or her bill or responded to your letters. Inquire whether there may be some questions regarding the bill. You may get responses about forgetting, hardships, or the fact that there are other bills to pay. It is important—whether you get legitimate reasons, excuses, or stalls—to be understanding while working toward a date when the patient will make a payment. Get a specific time and amount that you can then reiterate: "Then I can expect to receive one half of the outstanding balance by the 15th, and the rest the following month?" Conclude the call by indicating that the patient is free to call should he or she feel you can be of help, and that you are still available to the patient even though his or her account is in arrears.

If the plan is not adhered to, it is important to quickly follow up. Such reasons as "My husband has been out of work;" "We don't have the money;" "Things are too tight;" "I just began working at a new job" can all be responded to with understanding, while emphasizing a particular time within the week or at most within the month that payment will be expected. Many patients feel their insurance plan would or should pay for the procedures, and it is important to let the client know that very few insurance companies pay 100 percent of a mental health outpatient bill. Furthermore, it is important to underscore the fact that the arrangement between the client and the insurance company is one thing and between the client and you is another.

Sometimes clients attempt to stall by letting you know that the check has been mailed or by requesting that you send another statement. If this account has been outstanding for a while, stalls should be responded to more forcibly. Let the client know the importance of good credit and that if you don't hear from them within a specific period of time (usually two weeks) you will take the matter up with your attorney.

When it appears clear that you will not get paid for your service by a client then you need to consider one of the following procedures: referral to a collection agency, a lawyer, or Small Claims Court. Choosing a collection agency should be done with care. In addition to wanting to collect the fee, you have your reputation to consider as well. In general, experiences with collection agencies have not been particularly satisfactory. The attorney you have consulted for advice in setting up your practice will send a letter advising your client that if he or she does not pay within a certain period of time litigation will be brought on your behalf. The collection agency or attorney takes a large percentage of the money, usually one-third of what they collect.

The third alternative, which has been used rather successfully, is Small Claims Court. It requires a minimum amount of time to get on the docket, usually a few minutes to file papers, and, if you have a secretary or receptionist, this person usually can handle this aspect for you. The delinquent patient in my experience usually does not appear and thus loses by default and is ordered by the Court to pay the bill, or when he or she receives the summons to appear in Court, pays prior to the appearance date. Some clients even wait to see whether you will appear and then hand the bailiff your check. Most clients do not like to have judgments declared against them as this can affect their credit rating and their ability to borrow money in the future. Taking this step often will lead to quick payment or at least will create some communication with clients desiring the opportunity for setting up a schedule of payments.

## CONCLUDING COMMENTS

Some financial worksheets will bring this long but important chapter to a close. Although the items will vary from practitioner to practitioner and from locality to locality, they will give the mental health practitioner some general idea of what to expect when considering entering the world of private practice. The worksheets presented in Tables 2–2 and 2–3 are modified with the permission of Mark Lewin, who advises "Starting a business is exciting but scary. Starting one without doing one's homework is foolhardy. Those who rush into private practice fast, often repent at leisure. So start slowly and increase the probability of enjoying your professional practice" (1978, p. 74).

**Table 2–2** Financial Worksheet: Start-Up "One-Time" Costs

| *Item* | *Estimated Cost* |
|---|---|
| Rental security deposit | $________ |
| Initial professional supplies | ________ |
| Office furniture (including typewriter, phone answering device, desks, chairs, etc.) | ________ |
| Office supplies and expendables | ________ |
| Signs for door and building | ________ |
| Announcement promotional expenses | ________ |
| Telephone installation | ________ |
| Legal and accounting start-up costs | ________ |
| Cash for first month's "salary" (since there is likely to be a time lag between starting the practice and receiving initial payments of billings.) | ________ |
| TOTAL | $________ |

**Table 2–3** Financial Worksheet: Estimated Fixed and Variable Monthly Payments

| *Item* | *Estimated Expenses* |
|---|---|
| Salary or "draw" of practitioner | $______ |
| FICA (Social Security) | ______ |
| Secretarial and other wages | ______ |
| Secretarial FICA | ______ |
| State and federal taxes | ______ |
| Unemployment insurance | ______ |
| Office rent | ______ |
| Office cleaning and maintenance | ______ |
| Office supplies (pens, paper, stationery, typewriter ribbons, photocopying, etc.) | ______ |
| Professional supplies | ______ |
| Professional memberships, books, and journals | ______ |
| Continuing education and convention expenses | ______ |
| Postage | ______ |
| Telephone | ______ |
| Utilities | ______ |
| Travel expenses | ______ |
| Professional liability insurance | ______ |
| Medical insurance | ______ |
| Income protection insurance | ______ |
| Comprehensive fire, theft, office liability insurance | ______ |
| Life insurance | ______ |
| Professional services (legal and accounting) | ______ |
| Pension payments | ______ |
| Depreciation on furniture and office equipment | ______ |
| Miscellaneous (gifts, business lunches, charity, allowance for uncollectable bills, etc.) | ______ |
| TOTAL | $______ |

Choose the items that are applicable to you and then fill out the financial worksheets. This exercise will give you a good idea of how much money you will need to start your practice, and how much you will have to bill monthly to "stay in business." It might come as somewhat of a shock to consider that a full-time practitioner who wants an annual take-home salary of $30,000 must generate approximately $4,500 a month. This schedule of income and expenses includes some of the following major monthly expenses (using 1981 dollars):

| | |
|---|---|
| Income | $2,500 |
| Rent | 250 |
| Taxes | 650 |
| Secretary | 300 |

The practitioner whose practice requires a monthly billing of $4,500 will need to have approximately 33 billable contacts per week at $45.00 an hour. The lower the fee the more hours, and, conversely, the higher the fee the fewer the hours needed to reach this plan for income. Of course, these figures will vary depending on local conditions.

## SUMMARY

Major business decisions that the independent practitioner needs to consider when setting up the office were covered in this chapter. The following seven areas were highlighted:

- Situating your office
- Utilizing your office
- Structuring your business practice
- Owning or renting
- Furnishing
- Choosing professional materials
- Accounts receivable

Chapter 3

# More Business Headaches: Documentation and Record Keeping

# 3

The wish to escape regulatory red tape is often a major factor that propels practitioners to enter private practice. Federal and state agencies, accreditation review boards, third-party payers such as Medicaid, Medicare, private insurance companies, county health boards, and public funding agencies (United Way/Community Chest) all have a say in the way agencies such as community mental health centers run their businesses. In turn, these regulatory agencies directly and indirectly have a major influence on the mental health practitioner's work in private practice. As with the fortress that turns into a jail, so the need for documentation and concern for consumer rights can haunt the supposed refuge of the private practitioner.

In the previous chapter we considered record keeping from a financial point of view: accounts receivable and expenses payable. Now we will explore the importance of clinical record keeping, which is much more than keeping good treatment progress notes. Whether for public or private practice, we are now seeing an increased push for greater accountability of mental health professionals.

When the practitioner thinks about record keeping, the following has to be considered: regulatory-related aspects of record keeping, content-related aspects of record keeping, and retrieval-related aspects of record keeping.

## REGULATORY-RELATED ASPECTS OF RECORD KEEPING

There are a myriad number of rules or regulations governing who may perform what record keeping services (in a community agency only trained and certified record librarians can have access to medical records), the type of information that must appear in a record (documentation of physical ailments related to mental condition), with whom the content of the record can be shared (confidentiality), and whether the client has awareness of the procedures to be performed (informed consent).

Confidentiality, patient rights, and review boards (both peer and utilization ) are three regulatory-related aspects of record keeping that currently impact on the private practitioner. They often involve "nonproductive" time. It is easy to become careless in recognizing and attending to these areas.

### Confidentiality

The confidentiality of a client's record is intricately related to the integrity of the doctor-patient relationship. Every precaution must be taken to preserve confidentiality:

- Records must be kept in a locked filing cabinet.
- Discussion and disclosures regarding clients should be refrained from until specific permission is obtained from the client, preferably in writing.
- If material is used from a case, the demographic information should be disguised, and permission should be obtained from your client.
- Information that is disclosed should be reported fairly; information should be conveyed only if necessary to accomplish the purpose for which it was released.
- Confidentiality is basic for the client's protection.

Breaches of confidentiality are unethical and in states where there are laws governing confidentiality, illegal.

Mental health practitioners are constantly requesting and having others make requests for information. A written consent form is an integral part of consideration regarding patient's confidentiality. Key elements include:

- name of person to whom the disclosure is to be made (or agency or both)
- name of person about whom information is being disclosed
- purpose of the disclosure
- extent of the disclosure
- time limit of the disclosure
- ability to revoke disclosure

One example of a disclosure form is presented in Exhibit 3–1.

**Exhibit 3–1** Consent for Release of Information Form

Stanley Kissel, Ph.D.
123 Park Street
Rochester, New York

*CONSENT FOR RELEASE OF INFORMATION*

Permission is hereby given to:

______________________________________________

(Name of organization or individual obtaining or communicating information)

(To obtain information from) or (To communicate with): *CIRCLE ONE OR BOTH*

______________________________________________

(Name of organization or individual releasing or communicating information)

Regarding:

______________________________________________

The purpose or need for releasing this data shall be:

______________________________________________

(Specific purpose or need for the disclosure)

This authorization is limited to:

______________________________________________

(Extent or nature of information to be disclosed)

I hereby authorize the release of the above information from my record (child's record). I understand that the information to be released from my record (child's record) is confidential and protected from disclosure. I also understand that I have the right to cancel my permission to release information from my record (child's record) at any time before it is released. I also understand that my Consent for Release of Information will expire 90 days from this date if not acted upon prior to that time.

| | |
|---|---|
| ______________________ | ______________________ |
| Signature of Witness | Signature of minor if applicable |
| ______________________ | ______________________ |
| Date Signed | Signature |
| ______________________ | ______________________ |
| Expiration Date | Address |

Even in states that do not have sanctioned confidentiality—there are 16 states that do not have privileged communication status (Stetler & Moritz, 1962)—professional associations have incorporated statements regarding confidentiality into their code of ethics.

> A physician may not reveal the confidence entrusted in him in the course of medical attendance or the deficiencies he may see in the character of patients unless he is required to do so by law or unless it becomes necessary to protect the welfare of the individual or the community. (Principles of Medical Ethics, 1957)

The American Psychological Association Code of Ethical Standards (1977) states as follows:

> Safeguarding information about an individual that has been obtained by the psychologist in the course of his teaching or practice or investigation is a primary obligation of the psychologist. Such information is not communicated to others unless certain important conditions are met.
>
> A. Information received in confidence is revealed only after the most careful deliberation and when there is clear and imminent danger to a person or society and then only to appropriate professional workers or public authorities.
>
> B. Information obtained in clinical or consulting relationship, or evaluative data concerning children, students, employees and others, are discussed only for professional purposes and only with persons clearly concerned with the case. Written and oral reports should present only data germane to the purpose of the evaluation and every effort should be made to avoid undue invasion of privacy.
>
> C. Clinical and other materials are used in classroom teaching and writing only when the identities of the persons involved are adequately disguised.
>
> D. The confidentiality of professional communications about individuals is maintained. Only when the originator and other persons involved give their expressed permission is a confidential professional communication shown to the individual concerned. The psychologist is responsible for informing the client of the limits of the confidentiality.
>
> E. Only after explicit permission has been granted is the identity of research subjects published. When data have been published without permission the psychologist assumes responsibility for adequately disguising their sources.

F. The psychologist makes provisions for the maintenance of confidentiality in the preservation and ultimate disposition of confidential records.

Since the consequences of an unwarranted release of confidential information are ambiguous yet serious, the clinician must be very cautious. Assure yourself that the person you are informing is entitled to the information, have your client's permission to release the information, and if you have doubts, consult your attorney.

Privileged communication, informed consent, and patients' rights, including their right to review their records, are three other regulatory issues related to confidentiality.

### Privileged Communication

While confidentiality more often than not relates to a practitioner's ethical duty to keep secret the information obtained in a clinical relationship, the communication from patient to doctor becomes privileged only by state law. The state legislature has to pass a bill that such information revealed in the professional doctor-patient relationship may not be disclosed in legal proceedings without the patient's consent. Privileged communication laws differ from state to state. Some states give privileged communication to physicians but not to nonmedical mental health practitioners. Local and state mental health boards would be a helpful resource in determining whether the law in your state confers a privileged status to your profession. The clinician is, after all, the patient's personally selected representative.

When law requires the disclosure, as in child abuse, the clinician's duty is clear: to obey the law. In the more typical case the practitioner has to decide:

- whether the patient actually would carry out a threat he or she has made
- whether the patient can be persuaded to change his or her plans
- whether the patient will agree to have a responsible family member notified.
- whether concern for public safety requires an immediate disclosure.

If you refrain from acting because you believe that the patient is only playing a game in fantasy, you are taking a risk; but, then, working with the mentally ill, emotionally disturbed, and behaviorally maladaptive is full of risks. The practitioner unwilling to take them had better move back to public practice or perhaps into another profession.

## Informed Consent

Informed consent does not serve only the purpose of getting the patient's written approval for disclosing information; informed consent also makes the patient aware of the procedures involved in disclosing information, as well as the possible consequences of those procedures. Generally, clinicians inform patients about what to expect from psychotherapy or a diagnostic evaluation in a rather casual fashion: at times in response to a particular question or as a helpful suggestion to parents who are concerned about how to prepare their child.

Filling out a form, such as the one shown in Exhibit 3–2, is one suggested approach to informing your clients about what they can expect:

---

**Exhibit 3–2** Treatment Plan Form

*TREATMENT PLAN*

Name: ______________________________

Address: ______________________________

Problem:

Objective:

Treatment Modality:

Client's Signature: ______________________________

Clinician's Signature: ______________________________

Date Signed: ______________________

When filling out the treatment plan form with your client, list each problem separately. For each problem used, specify an objective; and for each objective specify a treatment and possible side effects.

In order for the patient's informed consent for treatment to be effective, the patient has to have adequate information about the treatment, available alternatives, and the *collateral* risks. Until recently the prevailing view was that if psychotherapy is not helpful, at least it is not harmful. More and more clinicians have begun questioning this point of view. In the past, courts followed the general rule of "professional standards of care" in determining what must be disclosed to a patient. The professional was thus given great leeway in deciding what was in the patient's best interests. However, in 1979 the Supreme Court of Oklahoma stated:

> We decline to adopt a standard based on professional standards. We therefore hold the scope of a physician's communication must be measured by his patient's need to know enough to enable him to make an intelligent choice. In other words, full disclosure of all *material risk,* incident to treatment, must be made.
>
> There is no right line separating the material from the immaterial: it is a question of fact. A risk is material if it would be likely to affect the patient's decision. When non-disclosure of a particular risk is open to debate, the issue is for the finder of facts. (*Scott* v. *Bradford*, 606, P.2d 554, Supreme Court Oklahoma 1979).

Patient records, once the property of the professional, have become the patient's to inspect, to copy, and to challenge. When a patient is unable to have certain portions of the record deleted or corrected, any written statement disputed in the record must be disclosed whenever that portion of the record is disclosed. Furthermore, the client now has the right to contest clinical records in a court of law.

## Consumer Rights

Title 5 of Public Law 96-398, which was passed in October 1980, created mental health rights and advocacy. The patient's bill of rights is presented in Exhibit 3–3.

**Exhibit 3–3** The Patient's Bill of Rights (PL 96-398)

TITLE V—MENTAL HEALTH RIGHTS AND ADVOCACY

BILL OF RIGHTS

State laws, review and revision. 42 USC 9501.

SEC. 501. It is the sense of the Congress that each State should review and revise, if necessary, its laws to ensure that mental health patients receive the protection and services they require; and in making such review and revision should take into account the recommendations of the President's Commission on Mental Health and the following:

(1) A person admitted to a program or facility for the purpose of receiving mental health services should be accorded the following:

Appropriate treatment and related services.

(A) The right to appropriate treatment and related services in a setting and under conditions that—

(i) are the most supportive of such person's personal liberty; and

(ii) restrict such liberty only to the extent necessary consistent with such person's treatment needs, applicable requirements of law, and applicable judicial orders.

Individualized written treatment or service plan.

(B) The right to an individualized, written, treatment or service plan (such plan to be developed promptly after admission of such person), the right to treatment based on such plan, the right to periodic review and reassessment of treatment and related service needs, and the right to appropriate revision of such plan, including any revision necessary to provide a description of mental health services that may be needed after such person is discharged from such program or facility.

Service planning, participation.

(C) The right to ongoing participation, in a manner appropriate to such person's capabilities, in the planning of mental health services to be provided such person (including the right to participate in the development and periodic revision of the plan described in subparagraph (B)), and, in connection with such participation, the right to be provided with a reasonable explanation, in terms and language appropriate to such person's condition and ability to understand, of—

(i) such person's general mental condition and, if such program or facility has provided a physical examination, such person's general physical condition;

(ii) the objectives of treatment;

(iii) the nature and significant possible adverse effects of recommended treatments;

(iv) the reasons why a particular treatment is considered appropriate;

**Exhibit 3–3** continued

(v) the reasons why access to certain visitors may not be appropriate; and

(vi) any appropriate and available alternative treatments, services, and types of providers of mental health services.

(D) The right not to receive a mode or course of treatment, established pursuant to the treatment plan, in the absence of such person's informed, voluntary, written consent to such mode or course of treatment, except treatment—

(i) during an emergency situation if such treatment is pursuant to or documented contemporaneously by the written order of a responsible mental health professional; or

(ii) as permitted under applicable law in the case of a person committed by a court to a treatment program or facility.

Experimentation, right of nonparticipation.

(E) The right not to participate in experimentation in the absence of such person's informed, voluntary, written consent, the right to appropriate protections in connection with such participation, including the right to a reasonable explanation of the procedure to be followed, the benefits to be expected, the relative advantages of alternative treatments, and the potential discomforts and risks, and the right and opportunity to revoke such consent.

Freedom from restraint or seclusion.

(F) The right to freedom from restraint or seclusion, other than as a mode or course of treatment or restraint or seclusion during an emergency situation if such restraint or seclusion is pursuant to or documented contemporaneously by the written order of a responsible mental health professional.

Humane treatment.

(G) The right to a humane treatment environment that affords reasonable protection from harm and appropriate privacy to such person with regard to personal needs.

(H) The right to confidentiality of such person's records.

Records, right of access.

(I) The right to access, upon request, to such person's mental health care records, except such person may be refused access to—

(i) information in such records provided by a third party under assurance that such information shall remain confidential; and

(ii) specific material in such records if the health professional responsible for the mental health services concerned has made a determination in writing that such access would be detrimental to such person's health, except that such material may be made available to a similarly licensed health professional selected by such person and such health professional may, in the exercise of professional judgment, provide such person with access to any or all parts of such material or otherwise disclose the information contained in such material to such person.

(J) The right, in the case of a person admitted on a residential or inpatient care basis, to converse with others privately, to have convenient and reasonable access to the telephone and mails, and to see visitors during regularly scheduled hours, except that, if a mental health professional treating such person determines that denial of access to a particular visitor is necessary for treatment purposes, such

*(continues)*

**Exhibit 3–3** continued

mental health professional may, for a specific, limited, and reasonable period of time, deny such access if such mental health professional has ordered such denial in writing and such order has been incorporated in the treatment plan for such person. An order denying such access should include the reasons for such denial.

(K) The right to be informed promptly at the time of admission and periodically thereafter, in language and terms appropriate to such person's condition and ability to understand, of the rights described in this section.

Grievance assertions.

(L) The right to assert grievances with respect to infringement of the rights described in this section, including the right to have such grievances considered in a fair, timely, and impartial grievance procedure provided for or by the program or facility.

Rights protection service, right of access.

(M) Notwithstanding subparagraph (J), the right of access to (including the opportunities and facilities for private communication with) any available—

(i) rights protection service within the program or facility;

(ii) rights protection service within the State mental health system designed to be available to such person; and

(iii) qualified advocate;

for the purpose of receiving assistance to understand, exercise, and protect the rights described in this section and in other provisions of law.

(N) The right to exercise the rights described in this section without reprisal, including reprisal in the form of denial of any appropriate, available treatment.

(O) The right to referral as appropriate to other providers of mental health services upon discharge.

(2)(A) The rights described in this section should be in addition to and not in derogation of any other statutory or constitutional rights.

Records, rights and accessability after discharge.

(B) The rights to confidentiality of and access to records as provided in subparagraphs (H) and (I) of paragraph (1) should remain applicable to records pertaining to a person after such person's discharge from a program or facility.

Right of admission to program or facility.

(3)(A) No otherwise eligible person should be denied admission to a program or facility for mental health services as a reprisal for the exercise of the rights described in this section.

(B) Nothing in this section should—

(i) obligate an individual mental health or health professional to administer treatment contrary to such professional's clinical judgment;

(ii) prevent any program or facility from discharging any person for whom the provision of appropriate treatment, consistent with the clinical judgment of the mental health professional primarily responsible for such person's treatment, is or has become impossible as a result of such person's refusal to consent to such treatment;

(iii) require a program or facility to admit any person who, while admitted on prior occasions to such program or facility, has repeatedly frustrated the purposes of such admissions by withholding consent to proposed treatment; or

(iv) obligate a program or facility to provide treatment services to any person who is admitted to such program or facility solely for diagnostic or evaluative purposes.

**Exhibit 3–3** continued

(C) In order to assist a person admitted to a program or facility in the exercise or protection of such person's rights, such person's attorney or legal representatives should have reasonable access to— **Records and information, accessability.**

(i) such person;

(ii) the areas of the program or facility where such person has received treatment, resided, or had access; and

(iii) pursuant to the written authorization of such person, the records and information pertaining to such person's diagnosis, treatment, and related services described in paragraph (1)(I).

(D) Each program and facility should post a notice listing and describing, in language and terms appropriate to the ability of the persons to whom such notice is addressed to understand, the rights described in this section of all persons admitted to such program or facility. Each such notice should conform to the format and content for such notices, and should be posted in all appropriate locations. **Notice.**

(4)(A) In the case of a person adjudicated by a court of competent jurisdiction as being incompetent to exercise the right to consent to treatment or experimentation described in subparagraph (D) or (E) of paragraph (1), or the right to confidentiality of or access to records described in subparagraph (H) or (I) of such paragraph, or to provide authorization as described in paragraph (3)(C)(iii), such right may be exercised or such authorization may be provided by the individual appointed by such court as such person's guardian or representative for the purpose of exercising such right or such authorization. **Incompetent persons.**

(B) In the case of a person who lacks capacity to exercise the right to consent to treatment or experimentation under subparagraph (D) or (E) of paragraph (1), or the right to confidentiality of or access to records described in subparagraph (H) or (I) of such paragraph, or to provide authorization as described in paragraph (3)(C)(iii), because such person has not attained an age considered sufficiently advanced under State law to permit the exercise of such right or such authorization to be legally binding, such right may be exercised or such authorization may be provided on behalf of such person by a parent or legal guardian of such person. **Incapacitated persons.**

(C) Notwithstanding subparagraphs (A) and (B), in the case of a person admitted to a program or facility for the purpose of receiving mental health services, no individual employed by or receiving any remuneration from such program or facility should act as such person's guardian or representative.

### Peer Review

It has been suggested that in a few years some form of peer review may be requested by insurance carriers in all 50 states (APA Monitor, January, 1981). Psychologists whose clients are insured by Champus will be requested to complete special treatment reports and submit them with claims at specific treatment intervals for peer review. Aetna, Equitable Life, Provident Mutual, Prudential, and New England Mutual Insurance companies have all expressed interest in peer review for mental health services.

Clinicians should be prepared to supply reviews and information so their colleagues can make educated judgments as to the necessity and adequacy of care being supplied to clients. If practitioners document their work, including the initial evaluation, psychological testing, consultation or treatment (consistent with the principles and guidelines that will be suggested in the following section on content-related aspects of record keeping), they should have minimum difficulty with peer review committees.

## CONTENT-RELATED ASPECT OF RECORD KEEPING

In the previous section we learned that federal, state, and professional regulatory agencies and boards have made clinical records more accessible to public scrutiny. A related issue is the recognition that clear documentation of your clinical work is an important component of proper patient care—whether you see your patient for the first time during an initial evaluation, provide consultation to a community agency, or have continued involvement with a client in psychotherapy. In the final analysis, good record keeping is necessary and serves as the basis of systematic review and evaluation of your patient's progress.

### Initial Evaluation

It is often helpful to develop a standardized approach to initial evaluations. This can save time, minimize the possibility of omitting relevant information, and foster a helpful flow during these very important early patient contacts. The following eight steps make for easy documentation of your initial evaluative sessions, provide basic information that will be necessary to get your bills paid, and form the basis of reasonable and responsible treatment plans.

*Step. 1: Client Identification*

The following information should be included:

- name
- date of birth
- sex
- address
- any specific identifying features such as body build, gait, posture, dress, cleanliness, scars, etc.

*Step. 2: Source and Reason for Referral*

Include the name of the person or agency referring the client and those concerns, complaints, symptoms, and problems that brought the client to your attention. Some clinicians provide their referral sources with a list of possible problems to check off, others have their patients fill out a brief symptom checklist, and yet others inquire "What brought you to see me today?"

*Step. 3: Presenting Circumstances*

It depends on whether the patient is a child, an adult, or a family as to what will be included in this section. The clinician will attempt to gain a history of the complaints, including such things as:

- onset
- frequency
- previous ways of handling the problem
- previous mental illness or previous mental health consultations for this or related problems

Significant background information should be noted on such issues as:

- parental relationships
- marital adjustment
- vocational history
- childhood fears, or difficulties

If the patient is a child, inquire about:

- sibling relationships
- education
- the mother's pregnancy, delivery, and the child's developmental milestones.

*Step. 4: Clinical Observation/Test Findings*

When your patient is an adult, a formal mental status examination should be recorded. If the patient is a child, describe pertinent information from your interview. If you have performed psychological testing, record an integrated summary of your findings and a listing of the tests administered.

Many nonmedically oriented health practitioners are not familiar with a mental status examination. The following sections illustrate the major areas that make up a mental status examination. Some of this information may already be available. The intent is not to present material that all practitioners must already know. Rather it is a guide for organizing that knowledge, along with a checklist for reviewing the inclusiveness of your procedures.

*Characteristics of Talk*

The manner in which the patient talks enables us to appreciate difficulties with his or her thought processes. It is desirable to obtain a verbatim sample of the stream of speech to illustrate psychopathologic disturbances.

Describe the speech—soft or loud, stuttering, hesitant, accent, enunciation (use test phrases like "Methodist Episcopal," "liquid linoleum," "third royal riding artillery brigade").

Note speed and quantity—rate of talk and if it varies with special topics, or affects. Observe any relationship with motor activity, and whether the patient is over-talkative or under-talkative. Any delay in answering questions due to intellectual deficiency, fear, suspicion, or language difficulty should be differentiated from retardation.

Note whether the patient's talk is coherent or incoherent. Does he or she proceed logically toward definite goal ideas or is his or her thinking illogical, vague, and loosely organized? With a disorder of logical association of ideas there may be scattering of the stream of speech (a degree of incoherence in which all associative continuity is lost.) Where this is extreme, it is often referred to as "verbigeration," with the final product amounting to a "word salad" replete with neologisms (self-invented words or phrases.)

Note the presence of any of the following:

- *Blocking*—sudden stoppage in the stream of talk for no apparent external (environmental) reason and without the patient being able to account for the block. It is usually due to the sudden appearance of affectively charged topics of preoccupation, or interference by delusional thoughts or hallucinatory phenomena.
- *Circumstantiality*—much unnecessary detail given spontaneously. Person is voluble, speech lacks incisiveness, but the goal is ultimately reached.
- *Perseveration*—repetition of speech (or movement) despite patient's efforts to produce a new answer.
- *Flight of Ideas*—overproductivity of talk that is continuous but the ideas are fragmentary. The connections between the parts of speech are often determined by chance associations between the fragments. A certain coherence or loose associative relation is present but the direction of talk is influenced by chance stimuli from internal or external sources. The original goal (answering a question) is lost sight of and not attained. With flight of ideas one may see punning, rhyming, clang association (on the basis of similar sounds), and distractibility.
- *Mutism*—no response at all even though the patient may give indications of contact and an awareness of the environment.
- *Substitution*—the use of related words approximating the definitive term (e.g., "I have *menu* three times a day" when "meals" would be the definitive term).

*Emotional State: Affective Reactions*

It may be extremely difficult to evaluate a patient's emotional state. It is necessary to obtain information on both the patient's subjective experiences as well as the objective expressions of his or her affective reaction.

Objectively, one should observe facial expression, motor behavior, the presence of tears, flushing, sweating, tachycardia, tremors, respiratory irregularities, and states of excitement, fear, and depression.

Much valuable information may be obtained by noting the relationship between the patient and the examiner. Attitudes of hostility, suspiciousness, or flirtatiousness, a desire for bodily contact, or outspoken criticisms should be noted.

Subjective data is obtained through the use of nonleading questions such as, "How are you feeling?" If the patient replies by using such general terms as "nervous," he or she should be asked to describe how the "nervousness" shows itself, how it affects him or her. Such words may mean different things to different individuals.

Under ordinary circumstances the affect varies with the situation and the subject under discussion. The psychiatrically ill patient is apt to have a persistent emotional trend based upon his or her particular emotional disorder. If a particular emotional trend is established, such as depression, further inquiry should attempt to elicit the depth and intensity and persistence of this emotional reaction. The patient should be asked if he or she has been crying or has felt like crying, whether he or she feels discouraged, or whether he or she has been troubled by thoughts of hurting himself or herself.

It is desirable to record a verbatim reply to questions concerning the patient's mood. The relationship between mood and the content of thought is of particular significance. There may be a wide divergence between what the patient says or does on the one hand and the patient's emotional state as expressed objectively in his or her face, or attitudes, or in relation to the subjective expressions of his or her emotional feelings.

One should note whether an intense emotional response accompanies the discussion of specific topics. *Shallowness* or *flattening of the affect* is indicated by an insufficiently intense emotional display in association with ideas or situations that ordinarily would call for a more adequate response.

*Dissociation* or *disharmony* between affect and thought content is often indicated by a qualitatively inappropriate emotional response, such as smiling or silly behavior when the attitude should be one of concern, anxiety, or sadness.

The evaluation of emotional reactions may be made even more difficult by the tendency some patients may demonstrate toward *simulation* or play acting. Patients who are trying to cover up a deep depression may feign cheerfulness and good spirits. The reverse may also be true. It may be necessary to refer to the nurse's notes or to observations made by other members of the psychiatric staff concerning the patient when he or she is not aware of being observed.

The patient's emotional reactions may be constant or may fluctuate during the examination. An attempt should be made to specify the ease or readiness with which such changes occur in response to pleasant or unpleasant stimuli. The degree or intensity of these affective responses should be specified in relative terms such as the following: composed, complacent, frank, friendly, playful, teasing, silly, cheerful, boastful, elated, grandiose, ecstatic; tense, worried, anxious, pessimistic, sad, perplexed, bewildered, gloomy, depressed, frightened; aloof, superior, disdainful, distant, defensive, suspicious; irritable, resentful, hostile, sarcastic, angry, furious; indifferent, resigned, apathetic, dull, affectless.

The term *emotional deterioration* is often used to indicate an easily suggestible state with a progressive failure to show a normal emotional response.

However, this term is too general and it is best to specify instances indicating the patient's affective reactions.

*Content of Thought: Special Preoccupations and Experiences*

Describing the spontaneous trend of thought, noting the main topics of complaint and preoccupation, is of particular importance. This may be elicited by asking the patient questions such as, "Have you been ill or troubled in any way?" "Do you have any difficulties that you complain of?" The questions should be neutral and simple and serve primarily to get the patient started talking rather than to direct his or her trend of thought. If the patient is extremely verbose or definitely incoherent, it may be necessary to direct him with more specific questions. This should be avoided if possible.

Once an appropriate topic has been introduced by the patient, the examiner may then elicit further details by using carefully phrased questions. It is often easy for a patient to start with a discussion of physical complaints and from there lead into the realm of emotional disturbances.

Delusions of *reference* or *persecution* in which the patient has the delusion of being the object of environmental attention may be brought out by some of the following questions:

- "How have others been treating you?"
- "Do people like you?"
- "Have you ever been watched or spied upon or singled out for special attention?"
- "Do others have it in for you?"
- "What do they say or do?"

Delusions of *alien control* (passivity), feelings of being under the control or guidance of an external force for good or ill, are manifestations of abnormal submissiveness to internal needs or demands that are disowned and subsequently projected. The examiner may ask:

- "Do you ever feel your thoughts or actions are under any outside influences or control?"
- "How do you become aware of it?"
- "Have you had any unusual experiences?"
- "Have you ever been hypnotized?"
- "Is your mind controlled by thought waves, electricity, or radio waves?"
- "Have you ever felt thoughts in your mind that were not your own?"
- "Are you able to influence others, to read their minds, or to put thoughts in their minds?"

The patient may express delusions involving strange experiences, fixed ideas of having had strange, bizarre, or mystical experiences. They may be vaguely or vividly described.

- "Have you received strange messages?"
- "Have you been in communication with Christ or the Blessed Virgin?"
- "Have you received any messages from Heaven?"

*Nihilistic* delusions are those in which the patient more or less completely denies reality and existence. He or she states that nothing exists—everything is lost, or he or she may deny the existence of parts of his or her body, such as "I have no head, no stomach," or I cannot die; I will live to eternity."

Delusions of *self-depreciation* are often seen in connection with severe depression. The patient describes feelings of unworthiness, sinfulness, ugliness, emitting obnoxious odors, or that because of being unworthy or sinful he or she will be punished, tortured, or that people are making derogatory remarks about him or her. These may be brought out by asking:

- "Have you tended to feel yourself responsible, or to blame yourself, for your illness, difficulties, or present situation?" "Why?"

Delusions of *grandeur* may be associated with elated states, such as delusions of great wealth, strength, power, sexual potency, or identification with a famous person or even the Lord.

*Somatic* delusions, delusions of having cancer, lues, obstructed bowels, leprosy, or some imaginary disease should be distinguished from a preoccupation or overawareness of normal, visceral, or peripheral sensations. The patient may have a definite physical disease yet may misinterpret symptoms ordinarily associated with that disease.

*Hallucinations* are false sensory impressions without any external basis in fact. The examiner should try to elicit the source of the projection, for example, whether the patient hears voices coming from outside or inside his or her head. The clarity, distinctness, and intensity of the perception should be noted. Ordinarily, one notes hallucinations in relation to the senses (auditory, visual, olfactory, gustatory, tactile). Unless a patient is obviously hallucinating, one should be tactful in approaching the patient for evidences of hallucinatory phenomena:

- "Are you sensitive to noise?"
- "Do the noises in your head or ears disturb you?"

- "Do you have a vivid imagination?"
- "Tell me what happened."
- "Do you hear your own thoughts as if a voice were speaking?"

In the *visual* sphere one might ask:

- "Do you dream vividly?"
- "Do you ever have such visions when you are awake?"
- "Have you seen anything unusual?"

Patients may complain of a feeling of *unreality* in which the outside environment or realities seem to have changed:

- "Do things seem natural or real to you?"
- "Do people, trees, etc., look as they always have to you?"

A state of *depersonalization* refers to the feelings of change in, or loss of reality of, the self or of the emotions:

- "Do you feel natural?"
- "Are you aware of any change in yourself?"
- "Does your body feel changed or unreal or strange?"

*Obsessions,* insistent thoughts recognized as arising from the self, usually are regarded by the patient as absurd and relatively meaningless, yet they persist despite the patient's endeavors to rid himself or herself of them.

- "Do you have any thoughts you can't get rid of?"
- "Do you find yourself thinking of things and can't stop or are you ever aware of thoughts, words, phrases, or tunes going around in your mind and you find yourself unable to control them?"

*Compulsions* are repetitive acts performed through some inner need or drive and are thought to arrive against the subject's wishes and produce feelings of tension and anxiety if omitted:

- "Do you feel compelled to do certain acts or perform certain rituals?"
- "Do they seem reasonable to you?"
- "Do you feel uncomfortable until they are done, even though you may know them to be foolish or unimportant?"

Among the common compulsions that are seen are repetitive hand washing, rituals for dressing in a certain order, locking and relocking doors repeatedly, tapping on all wooden objects a certain number of times, etc. One should inquire about the fluctuations in kind, intensity, also any possible meaning of the act, illogical fears of special objects or situations leading to the insistent avoidance of them, such as fears of trains, subways, elevators, close spaces, crowds, or open spaces (*phobias*).

Fantasies and daydreams are often difficult to elicit from the patient. This may be due to a lack of understanding on the part of the patient of what the examiner wants. More often the patient is reluctant to talk about them because he or she feels ashamed about their content. Questions such as the following may be helpful in getting the patient's train of thought:

- "Do you ever imagine yourself going through situations before you meet them?"
- "Do you ever have any thoughts as to what you would do if you were very powerful or rich?"
- "Just how would you change yourself or the world or both if you could?"

The patient's main preoccupation or content of thought often reveals significant dynamic factors either directly or in the form of projections that enable us to get some understanding of the development of the illness. Some attempt should be made to evaluate whether the emotional reaction is primary and the mental trend is secondary to the affective state or whether the reverse is true.

### *Orientation*

Note should be made of the patient's ability to grasp the significance of his or her immediate situation and the clearness of his or her conscious processes. Confusion, bewilderment, and clouding of consciousness may be related to toxic or organic factors much more frequently than to psychodynamic factors.

Orientation should be tested for time, place, person, and self. The patient should be asked questions concerning the day of the week, the time of day, the date, the name of the building he or she is in, the city in which he or she lives. It is also important to determine the patient's ability to recognize personnel such as nurses and physicians and whether the patient knows who he or she is.

One may introduce such matters by asking a question like "Have you kept track of the time? If so, what is today's date?" If the patient does not know, he or she should be asked to estimate approximately or to guess at an answer.

This will give some idea of how much disturbance there is in orientation. The patient's attention may wander; he or she may show a prolonged reaction time or a complete failure to grasp the significance of the question.

*Memory*

In a broad clinical sense *memory* implies the ability to recall past experiences. Memory defects may be related to a *lack of attention* to the experience, difficulties in *retention,* difficulties in *recall,* or any combination of these three factors.

It is clinically helpful to differentiate between immediate retention and recall, memory for the recent past and for the remote past. The examiner should determine whether the defect is variable or constant, circumscribed for a particular time period (amnesia) or more extensive, and whether or not the patient makes an attempt to fabricate memories to take the place of those he or she has forgotten (*confabulation*).

It is useful to introduce questions relating to memory by some general statement such as:

- "Has your memory been good?"
- "Have you had any difficulty in concentrating or in remembering what you read?"
- "Have you had any difficulty with telephone numbers, appointment times, etc?"

• *Recall of Remote Past Experiences*—This part of the examination may be used to obtain a review of the important chronological facts of the individual's life history. Among the questions to be asked are: the time and place of birth, various schools the patient attended, occupational history, date of marriage, number of children and their ages as well as their names, and chronological data relating to the patient's past illnesses.

• *Recall of Recent Past Experiences*—This portion of the examination may be used to review the development of the present illness and the events leading to hospitalization and treatment. The patient should be asked when he or she first felt ill or troubled, when he or she came to the hospital, when he or she had to quit work, which physicians and nurses he or she has met, and what examinations and treatment have been given.

• *Recall of Immediate Impressions*—Here one tests the function of retention, such as the patient's ability to retain a person's name a few minutes after the introduction. Or the patient may be given three unrelated facts, such as a person's name, a color, and a street address and then be asked to repeat them immediately, and then again after a five-minute interval. The examiner should record the patient's ability for the immediate repetition of digits, starting with three or four digits until the patient fails twice. The digits are read to the patient at the rate of approximately one per second without rhythmical spacing or vocal inflection. The numbers chosen should not be in their natural order and should not suggest historical dates or other combinations of numbers familiar to the patient.

• *General Grasp and Recall*—The patient is asked to read the following story and then immediately upon completion to repeat the gist of the story giving as many details as possible:

The Cowboy Story

> A cowboy from Arizona went to San Francisco with his dog, which he left at a friend's house while he purchased a new suit of clothes. Dressed in the new suit, he went back to the dog, whistled to him, called him by name, and patted him. The dog would have nothing to do with him in his new hat and coat, but gave a mournful howl. Coaxing had no effect, so the cowboy went away and donned his old garments. Then the dog immediately showed his wild joy at seeing his master as he thought he ought to be.

*General Intellectual Evaluation*

If formal intelligence test results are not available the following may be helpful:

• *General Information*—The patient may be asked to give the five largest cities in the United States, the capitals of various states, the dates of the principal wars in the United States and the issues involved, the names of the last four presidents, the governor of the state, and to define differences in abstract words such as "idleness" and "laziness," "poverty" and "misery," "character and reputation."

• *Calculation*—The patient is asked to subtract seven from one hundred and continue subtracting seven until he or she can go no further. The answers should be recorded carefully, including the time taken for the test. If the patient makes an error he or she should not be corrected but urged to go on. Tests of simple multiplication are given as well as simple arithmetical problems such as "If two apples cost five cents, how many apples can you buy for thirty-five cents?"

• *Reasoning and Judgment*—The patient's ability to correctly estimate and form opinions concerning external objective matters indicates his or her relative freedom from impairment of judgment. He or she may be asked the difference between a dwarf and a child or what he or she would do with a gift of $10,000. The examiner should be careful not to allow his or her own biased opinions to enter into the evaluation of the patient's reasoning ability.

*Step. 5: Medical Status*

In this section include:

- the name of your client's primary physician
- approximate date of last physical examination
- any specific physical ailments that might affect the client's emotional or mental condition
- any medication being taken

*Step. 6: Impression*

In this section include your diagnostic formulations, thoughts concerning possible etiology factors, notes about the kind of person the client is, some life circumstances and stresses that relate to the client's current state, and your thoughts about prognosis.

*Step. 7: Diagnosis*

Although many mental health practitioners are opposed to utilizing a diagnostic or medical model, it is a practical matter to be prepared to provide a diagnosis to third-party payers if you expect or want your client to be reimbursed for professional services. The diagnostic classification of psychopathology adopted by the American Psychiatric Association is the most widely used and accepted diagnostic system. The independent practitioner should have a copy of the *Diagnostic and Statistical Manual,* 3rd ed. (DSM III) (Washington, D.C. American Psychiatric Association, 1980) on his or her desk.

*Step. 8: Recommendations*

Basically your recommendations should match the appropriate resources to the client's difficulties:

- *Environmental Change*—Recommend such actions as institutionalization, out-of-home placement, change of school or resource room, etc.
- *Chemotherapy*—If appropriate, list type of medication and dosage or state to whom the patient should be referred for what type of condition.
- *Psychotherapy*—Specify the type: individual, group, or family, and frequency of visits.
- *Referral*—Recommendations can be made for further evaluation, or for another specialist.

### Progress Notes

Progress notes serve a number of functions for the clinician:

- reviewing information
- charting the progress of treatment
- mapping strategy for future sessions
- documenting sessions held
- providing material for defending self if sued

It is wise to record progress notes at the end of each session but no later than the end of the same day. The notes should be brief and make some reference to the major problems—even if to say "not discussed today," the relationship you have with your client, progress being made, and future planning. It is helpful to record progress notes chronologically, using three-ring paper, so that each note can be fastened to the patient's chart when filed.

The following is a sample progress note:

Frank A. Patient — August 1, 1980

Frank was seen for his regular appointment today. He continues to show strong obsessions, but the suicidal thoughts continue to be absent. He appears to have accepted my suggestion as to the defensive nature of these thoughts. Frank is not a suicidal risk.

Today, spent bulk of our time regarding his mother, who is going into hospital for surgery. He worries she'll die, abandon him, and he'll have to start growing up and taking care of himself. Some past memories, hostile and erotic, entering consciousness. Pursue these and try to relate them to problem of being assertive and expressing anger.

He still continues to be resistant to day hospital referral.

### Closing Summary

The summary can also be a special progress note. It should be brief but include a statement of the problem, duration or number of sessions held, outcome of the treatment and reason for termination, and any follow-up plans. Some sample closing summaries follow:

Mr. and Mrs. Smith, referred by Dr. Black, pediatrician, because of inability to control seven-year-old son, John. Boy showing temper tantrums and sibling rivalry, yells and punches four-year-old sister.

John seen for eight sessions during February-April and parents seen twice. Progress with temper tantrums, some improvement in sibling relationship. Parents feel better able to control selves and children, especially John.

Decided to terminate as parents wanted to try on their own without support. Call on as needed basis. Diagnosis: DSM-III - Axis I - 309.28. Adjustment Disorder with Anxious Mood.

Michael was evaluated during October of 1980 because he exhibited hyperactive behavior at home and in school. Ritalin 20 mg after breakfast and 10 mg after lunch to reduce activity level was introduced.

Michael was followed on a monthly basis. The Ritalin had to be increased from time to time so that most recently he was receiving 30 mg after breakfast and 20 mg after lunch and later in the afternoon. These increases were necessitated when he seemed to escape the control of the medication and became extremely overactive in school on lesser amounts. Early in 1981 he was tried for a brief period on Meclizine up to 25 mg b.i.d. because there were some suggestions that a cerebellar involvement in the hyperactivity was present. This did not prove to be too helpful. Several years ago he also received Mellaril, 10 mg. h.s. for a short period of time because of difficulties in going to sleep. The last contact with Michael and his father was on April 17, 1981. At that time he was reported to be doing optimally on the aforementioned regimen of Ritalin. He has been referred for psychoeducational testing to the Learning Disabilities Clinic. Diagnosis: Hyperactivity with minimal brain dysfunction.

## RETRIEVAL-RELATED ASPECT OF RECORD KEEPING

While practitioners are not necessarily cavalier in their approach to records, the fact remains that most clinicians relegate record keeping to second-class priority status. Daily as well as long-term patient care can be hampered by poor management of records. It is important for the practitioner to develop good record-keeping habits when establishing the practice. While large institutions such as hospitals, community mental health centers, and courts have instituted complex record-keeping systems with large staffs of record-keeping librarians and filing clerks, it is not necessary to be elaborate in order to be efficient. However, taking a few extra minutes can make all the difference in the world. You simply cannot store records in a cabinet and expect to alphabetize them one day when you have some free time.

There are basically two major ways of approaching records: numerically or alphabetically. The alphabetical system is fine when there are not very many records to handle, but as the records become more voluminous a numbering system makes more sense. A numerical system also provides easier access for expansion.

A system that is most appropriate for practitioners who over time will be successful and generate many records is a combination of the two. It's basically a unit numbering system. The patient is assigned a number and when the case is closed, a folder containing all relevant materials is filed numerically. The number assigned is a six-digit number: the first two at the left represent the year, the remainder represent filing numbers. For example, a record numbered 80-70-5 means the case, opened in 1980, would be filed in section 5, the 70th record.

Using the year permits an easy cleanout of records when they either get old or space becomes a premium. Many states have statutes that specify how long a patient's record must be held. For example, New York State requires that all children's records be held for seven years beyond their twenty-first birthday and adult records be held for a minimum of ten years. The practitioner who finds filing space at a premium might prefer to weed out records every three years, box them, and put them in a storage area.

Current records are filed alphabetically.

The third part of this filing system involves keeping index cards listing name, assigned number, address, referral sources, and closing date. These are kept in alphabetical order. This system makes it easy to store and retrieve information on current and closed records for clinical and marketing purposes.

## SUMMARY

Now that we have considered the why, where, and how of private practice, the next step is to let the community know about your interest to practice privately. The next two chapters will address this issue.

Chapter 4

# Relevant Marketing

# 4

Unlike doctors or lawyers, who are primary providers of care, the mental health specialist is a secondary provider of care. That is, the mental health practitioner is dependent upon others for referral of patients and clients for service. While it is important to develop good professional practices and strive for excellence in work, unless referral sources are aware of your services and your reputation, or have experienced your competent clinical services, you can expect to spend many pleasant hours with your fantasies.

Both full-time and part-time practitioners share the need to "market their wares," that is, to inform potential referral sources of their services. Most mental health practitioners' training and philosophical-scientific orientation champions the view that it is undignified, unprofessional, and, until recently, unethical to advertise for services.

Informing the public and other professionals in the community about your availability is in and of itself a bona fide service. For example, primary patient care providers such as pediatricians or internists can provide better care for their patients if they are acquainted with some mental health referral sources. Family medicine practitioners come in contact with all age levels in the family and the more varied their referral base, the better the ultimate quality of care they can provide for their patients.

In this and the next chapter we will consider some traditional strategies that have been used successfully and some innovative marketing strategies that are available to many mental health practitioners if they take the time to look and listen with their heads rather than their eyes and ears.

*The most important point is to stop being so timid about your approach to independent practice!*

## USING THE MAILS

### Announcements

An announcement that one is going into private practice can be ethically placed in local newspapers and sent to colleagues and members of other professions who are believed to be possible referral sources. We will consider newspaper advertisements later in this chapter. There is some question as to whether or not mailing announcements to colleagues and potential referral sources matters or is just an exercise in narcissism and a waste of economic resources. I believe that such a practice can be wasteful only if the practitioner fails to use the announcement as a first step in a systematic approach to getting to know and getting to be known by possible referral sources. In one step you will no longer be an unknown name!

Many practitioners are penny wise and pound foolish when it comes to announcement cards. Mailing announcements is costly, no question about it. There is the high cost of postage, the cost of printing, and the time involved in addressing envelopes. For these reasons it pays to choose announcement cards carefully and remember that your announcement is a way of making a statement about yourself. The stock, the color of paper and ink, the type of printing—whether engraved, thermo-engraved, letterpress, or offset—are aspects to consider.

The following are the essential elements of an announcement card, as shown in Figure 4–1:

1. Your name is the most important aspect of the card. It should stand out.
2. You are telling the referral source who may know you by your reputation as a public practitioner that you have opened up private offices.
3. You are now beginning to form your identity as having a subspecialty.
4. This is the location where you can be reached.
5. This is the telephone number where messages will get to you reliably and quickly.

### Business Cards

Since direct mail-order advertising is the most expensive form of advertising, if possible send more than one piece through the mail each time you do a mailing. Business cards, which are a relatively inexpensive item yet an important marketing tool, should also be considered when ordering announcement cards. The business card will reinforce your professionalism and provide something else to include in your initial mailing that will again bring your name to the attention of the possible referral source. Include a few business cards, the purpose of which should be mentioned in a cover letter, which is the third piece of information to include in your announcement mailing.

The copy for the business card should be kept to a minimum and provide such essential information as specialty, location, and phone number (see Figure 4–2). Business cards are usually 3½ by 2 inches, printed on a white stock with black ink. Beige cards with brown ink, however, are being used with greater frequency and are more attractive in appearance. Cards are usually printed in lots of 500 and the supply should last for quite a while. The cost varies from $15.00 to $50.00, depending on the quality of paper and the type of printing.

---

**Figure 4–1** A Sample Announcement Card

1. STANLEY KISSEL, Ph.D.

2. ANNOUNCES THE OPENING
OF A PRIVATE PRACTICE IN

3. CHILD AND ADOLESCENT PSYCHIATRY

4. 1425 PORTLAND AVENUE
ROCHESTER, NEW YORK

5. TELEPHONE 544-5220

**Figure 4–2** A Sample Business Card

TELEPHONE 544-5220 TELEPHONE 381-4700

STANLEY KISSEL, PH.D.

OFFICE HOURS
BY APPOINTMENT ONLY

1425 PORTLAND AVENUE
ROCHESTER, N. Y. 14621

### The Cover Letter

It is especially important for practitioners new to an area or those who are attempting to expand their referral base (as in transition from part-time to full-time practice) to include a cover letter with their announcements. The cover letter should be concise, personal, and include the following points:

- what is being sent
- why it is being sent
- your expectation of sharing patients in the future

It may be unreasonable to expect that as many as one hundred letters will be individually typed but it makes a good impression if the body of the letter is offset printed and the salutation, signature, date, and address are typed, thus giving the appearance of a more personal letter. Furthermore, this makes for a neat prosperous-appearing letter. There are, of course, other materials that can be included in the mailing but it is important to know how much your items weigh, being careful not to exceed the one-ounce postage allowance. Along with the personal letter, you can include reprints of any published work in the area that the referral source might be interested in and referral procedures and forms that you would like used. Many of these, however, are best left for a second mailing or for an in-person meeting. The following is an example of an introductory letter:

> Dear Dr. Referral:
> I am writing to tell you that I have recently moved into your area and have opened professional offices for the independent practice of psychology. I will be providing a broad range of psychological services to both children and their parents. Although my specialty is psychotherapy, I will also be providing psychological evaluations of children. I trust that these services may be of benefit to some of your patients. I have enclosed some business cards that might be of help and would be delighted to meet with you and discuss my services further.

## USING THE PHONE

The cover letter, an announcement card, and some business cards for use with possible referrals make up the initial announcement packet. The announcement packet will give you something to use as an icebreaker when calling a new referral source for a face-to-face meeting. This is an important next step in cultivating new sources of referrals. A luncheon meeting is often a good approach.

It is important when making the telephone contact to a possible referral source, who might be an attorney, a physician, an administrator at an agency such as a community mental health center, the head of the probation department, or members of the juvenile division of the police, that after identifying yourself you ask whether the person is available to speak with you. If you have sent the prospective referrant the announcement packet, mention this as it gives you the opportunity to reinforce your professional affiliation, the location of your office, and the fact that you'd like to get together so you can explain more clearly and in more detail the services you provide. Suggest a lunch-time meeting by asking whether or not it would be convenient; also give the referrant the opportunity to suggest a date and a particular place, thus making it possible for the referrant to suggest coming to his or her office. Many busy primary practitioners prefer to bring lunch and have such meetings at their office.

## MEETING IN PERSON

At the meeting it is important for you to clearly make known your services, emphasizing how your particular service might be different from similar services. For example, if you are affiliated with a group, state how the group can provide a full range of mental health services; if you are doing what agencies in the community do, emphasize your quick feedback and ease of communication. Let the prospective referrant know about your training, your orientation, and find out the preferred mode of feedback. Most important is to establish a format for referrals. Have available a number of business cards that you can leave. Many referrants like to give the business card to patients they refer. A good ploy, however, is not to present both business cards and referral forms but to send some of either in the mail. This gives you an opportunity to send a follow-up letter, which provides the possible referrant with yet another reminder about you. Indeed, even if you don't have anything to send, it is a good idea to follow up the luncheon with a note commenting on some points discussed and thanking the referrant for his or her time.

## USING THE MEDIA

### Newspapers

Newspapers are another good place for you to announce the opening of your private offices. The announcement for the newspaper can be similar to the one sent to professionals in the community. Since this announcement will be read by a less-informed population it should clearly spell out your area or areas of expertise. An announcement two columns wide by three inches would be sufficient. One much bigger may appear ostentatious and uneconomical. Remember, it is unethical to mention your professional affiliation with an association such as the American Psychological Association. Professional competency, which may be inferred by such a designation, is not a requirement for membership. However, it is appropriate and advisable to use your diplomate status if you have achieved that status.

In addition to using newspapers for announcements they can be enlisted in other ways to enhance your visibility. Mental health practitioners often present at scientific meetings, provide workshops, or give talks to PTAs and church groups. News releases detailing these presentations can be sent to the newspapers. Newspapers are often interested in this type of news, especially local and town newspapers, which have considerable space they need to fill. The release should be timely, informative, and clearly state that you are in the independent practice of psychology, social work, etc. The American Psychological Association's media guide lists a number of suggestions for relating to the media. One of the pieces included is from the Society for Neuroscience's *Guide to Effective Communication with the Media* (Miller, 1978). The section on special points relevant to newsprint follows and is reproduced with permission of the Society.

> The primary function of newspapers and news magazines is to provide information on "what's new" to a broad readership, but entertainment is also a consideration. The news must be presented simply and must be interesting enough to hold attention. *Science news will be read only if it is presented in a simple, direct, and graphic way, and it will be printed only if the editor believes that it will be read.* While the primary content is the printed word, a good photograph or diagram can occasionally be useful.

It is important to remember that the journalists are first and foremost surrogates for their readers. As such, the journalist's primary obligation is to news as he or she perceives it—not to the sensibilities of the scientist or the scientist's institution. Moreover, controversy and scandal are every journalist's meat—and even better if they can be found hidden in some ivory tower.

There are very different kinds of newspapers and news magazines, each of which takes pride in its individuality and unique qualities. The following is a rough categorization.

### *Large Dailies*

Large dailies would be "world" newspapers such as the *New York Times*, the *Times* (of London), the *Washington Post*, and the *Christian Science Monitor*. Since one of their functions is to record ongoing history, they attempt to report news in all subject categories, even the scholarly and technical, if the event has broad significance. But all stories must compete for available space. Thus, depending on the vagaries of politics, military conflict, or earthquakes, a news development involving science may or may not make publication.

Newspapers must have a specific event as the point of departure for most of their stories. Since yesterday's news is stale, the reporter is racing a deadline. Wherever possible, it is merciful to give the writer a news release in advance of a specific event such as a scientific meeting. The story can have a release date that will be honored. It is useful to find out the paper's deadline and to schedule press conferences accordingly or, better yet, to arrange their timing in advance with a reporter.

The large newspaper will occasionally publish a longer story that may or may not arise from an important news development. This feature story will review the subject area, providing background to recent developments, in an attempt to give a broader understanding of the field to the general reader. Such stories are generally preplanned and researched, including information from interviews, and may take days or weeks to prepare instead of the minutes or hours that the news story is allowed. Feature stories are short versions of the more leisurely and literary feature articles that appear in weekly or monthly magazines.

### *Medium-Sized and Small Dailies*

The majority of U.S. newspapers are medium-sized and small dailies. Their needs and the coverage they provide differ from those of the large metropolitan paper. Usually, they will not have a writer who specializes in science or medical topics; the writer assigned to a science story one day may cover a fire the next. Most of the world or national news coverage in such papers comes from the wire services. Local names and places are important to these papers, and their primary interest may be in clinical developments rather than basic research. A major story from the wire service about a scientific breakthrough in another part of the country may be ignored in favor of a lesser story coming from a local school or hospital and featuring the names of local scientists.

## Wire Services

A scientist may think he or she is talking to a small hometown newspaper in Oregon about small clinical studies, and the next thing that happens is that Mother calls from Maine with congratulations about the Nobel-quality work she read about in her *local* paper. This is the work of the wire services, the most powerful though least understood organ of American journalism.

Polls show that most Americans get their news from television, but most of the news they hear on television is generated by the wire services—at least anything from out of town. And frequently, these wire services—The Associated Press (AP), United Press International (UPI), and Reuters—get their underlying news from local papers. So, if you are talking for any print reporters, no matter how small the newspaper, no matter where you are, always consider that what you say may wind up in newspapers or on TV all over the country, maybe all over the world.

The scientist must take time to help the reporter get it right. The reporter may overemphasize clinical implications, trying to make page one with the work of a local scientist, or he or she may misunderstand the implications entirely. Frequently, a wire service will pick this story up, without checking back with the scientist, and it will get national exposure at perhaps four paragraphs' length. This is the perfect length for a newspaper to fill out a column, so be forewarned.

The wire services have their own competent science and medicine correspondents, but they are powerless to keep off the wire the small out-of-perspective story from a local bureau—often written by young, ambitious reporters looking for the big story to start them up the ladder.

## Large Circulation Weeklies

*Time, Newsweek, Parade,* and *U.S. News & World Report* are examples of large circulation weeklies. (The *National Enquirer* poses special problems. It is frankly sensational and the distortions generated here can produce real harm in patients looking for "cures." Unfortunately, it has such a large readership that one regrets seeing its reporters left exclusively to the less reliable sources they frequently use.) These publications cannot cover fast-breaking news the way the dailies do; they attempt to provide more in-depth coverage of events and trends in the world. Their reporters have somewhat more time to research their stories than do those for the dailies; sometimes an article can be several days or even several weeks in preparation. Because their resources and circulation are so large, their impact is powerful.

## News Periodicals for Physicians

There are a number of organs that attempt to update professionals on all the new developments in their field. *Medical World News, Medical Tribune, Hospital Practices,* and *AMA News* are examples. For the most part, readers are busy practitioners who can manage to stay current in their own specialities but need to be aware of what is new in all areas of medicine, including basic research. Stories of new developments are brief but provide enough data and names of individuals for the reader to follow up in the literature a story that is close to his or her needs. The occasional feature article gives more perspective. Writers for these publications are necessarily highly skilled professionals with special training in one or more branches of medicine. They attend professional meetings and cull professional journals for leads to news. These writers can take time to prepare excellent articles. They are writing for a sophisticated and influential audience. Nonetheless, their requirements are closer to those of a newspaper than to those of a technical scientific journal.

## Magazines and Books

Magazines that are not primarily oriented toward the news (e.g., *The New Yorker, Ladies' Home Journal, Cosmopolitan, Esquire)* will occasionally run a feature story on a scientific topic. The requirements for these stories are similar to those of feature stories in newspapers or Sunday supplements. Sometimes they are written by staff writers who have little background in science; at other times, a science writer may be commissioned to produce a specific story or, as a free-lance writer, may sell one to a magazine. There is more time for research, more opportunity to interview a number of different investigators, more chance to check facts and allow the scientist to check what has been written.

A popular science book must have the same level of simple clear exposition as the other printed media, but because of its greater length, it can deal with more complicated subject material in more detail. The writer has more time to research the material but unless there is some type of grant support, in the long run he or she must average a reasonable number of words per day in order to earn a living.

### A News Release Format

The American Psychological Association's media guide suggests the following news release format:

- Your name—Use your letterhead or type it clearly on top.
- "For release:"—Use a date to coincide with a speech or workshop, etc. and type it in the upper right. Use "for immediate release" when the time the information is conveyed to the general public is not a factor. Include the date the release is to be mailed.
- "For additional information:"—Contact person should be included in the upper right or at the bottom of the page. Supply name, address (for mail), phone number with area code (where someone will answer).
- Headline—Should be as short as possible, a brief condensation of the most important part of the story. Use words that generalize the first paragraph. Be judicious in using a cute or catchy headline.
- Paragraph 1—One or two sentences with as much of the who, what, where, when, why, and how as possible. Subject releases that try, for example, to stimulate coverage on an individual's research or a project can be a bit different but generally still follow this format.
- Paragraphs 2, 3, 4—Keep to one idea per paragraph. With few exceptions keep paragraph short. Print on both sides of the paper, if necessary. Double spacing is best, although single will do (with double spacing between paragraphs). If you can keep a long message on one side of a sheet of paper 8½ by 11, it is best.
- Last paragraph—Note any attributions, sources, and other miscellany here.
- Don't—summarize, editorialize, or prophesy.

Exhibit 4–1 presents one example of a release that incorporates the points discussed.

**Exhibit 4–1** Sample News Release

For more information, call:
Stanley Kissel, Ph.D.
Rochester Mental Health Center
544-1234

FOR IMMEDIATE RELEASE

TO:

The third Parent Education Power series is scheduled for consecutive Wednesday evenings beginning May 3. The meetings are sponsored by the Children and Youth Division of the Rochester Mental Health Center and will be held in the Main Conference Room at Rochester General Hospital.

In announcing the current series, Dr. Stanley Kissel, Coordinator of the Family Education Unit, said the aim of the program is to teach parenting skills by combining knowledge, skill, and confidence.

More and more parents, Dr. Kissel stated, find they are unable to cope. "When parents lose confidence in their ability to guide children, all members of society suffer," he said.

The Family Education Unit's goal will be to assist parents in dealing with parenting stresses, which are often compounded by other problems and insecurities. All families, Dr. Kissel said, could benefit by education and information about developing skills as parents.

On Wednesday, May 3, David Trachtman will speak on "Psychiatric Crisis and Emergency Services." Mr. Trachtman is coordinator of the Psychiatric Emergency Department at the Rochester General Hospital and Associate Director of the Children and Youth Division at the Rochester Mental Health Center. Mr. Trachtman has been instrumental in setting up psychiatric emergency services in Rochester.

Dr. Stanley Kissel will discuss with parents the "Ins and Outs of Child Psychotherapy" on May 10. Dr. Kissel co-authored the recently published "Human Resources for Troubled Children" and has taught courses on parent/child relationships and family therapy.

Brian Vandenberg, a developmental psychologist, will deal with "Expectations of the Parent-To-Be" in the session of May 17. Mr. Vandenberg is a contributor to the "Expectant Parent" series at Rochester General Hospital.

In the final session, May 24, Dr. Nelli Mitchell, Supervising Clinical Psychiatrist at the Rochester Mental Health Center, will discuss "Emotional Problems of Developmentally Disordered Children." Dr. Mitchell is also a clinical associate at the University of Rochester Medical School, and has helped many local agencies develop programs for developmentally disabled children.

All lectures will be held from 7:30 to 9:00 p.m. on the dates above. The public is invited to attend. A donation of $1 will be requested to cover expenses.

## A CONSCIOUSNESS-RAISING CAUTION

Professional organizations such as the American Psychological Association and the American Speech-Language-Hearing Association have become more sensitive to communication in written style that may reinforce questionable attitudes and assumptions about people and sex roles. We, as responsible professionals, need to take care that our written communications do not reinforce sexism. Exhibit 4–2 presents suggested guidelines for nonsexist language reprinted with the permission of the American Psychological Association:

---

**Exhibit 4–2** Guidelines for Nonsexist Language

| | I. Problems of Designation | |
|---|---|---|
| Examples of common usage | Consider meaning. An alternative may be better. | Comment |
| | A. Ambiguity of Referent | |
| 1. The *client* is usually the best judge of the value of *his* counseling. | The *client* is usually the best judge of the value of counseling. | *His* deleted. |
| | *Clients* are usually the best judges of the value of the counseling they receive. | Changed to plural. |
| | The best judge of the value of counseling is usually *the client.* | Rephrased. |
| 2. *Man's search* for knowledge has led *him* into ways of learning that bear examination. | The *search* for knowledge has led *us* into ways of learning that bear examination. | Rephrased, using first person. |
| | *People* have continually sought knowledge. The search has led them, etc . . . | Rewritten in two sentences. |
| 3. man, mankind | people, humanity, human beings, humankind, human species | In this group of examples, a variety of terms may be substituted. |

**Exhibit 4–2** continued

| | | |
|---|---|---|
| man's achievements | human achievements, achievements of the human species. | |
| the average man | the average person, people in general | |
| man a project | staff a project, hire personnel, employ staff | |
| manpower | work force, personnel, workers | |
| Department of Manpower | (No alternative.) | Official titles should not be changed. |
| 4. The use of experiments in psychology presupposes the mechanistic nature of *man.* | The use of experiments in psychology presupposes the mechanistic nature of the *human being.* | Noun substituted. |
| 5. This interference phenomenon, called learned helplessness, has been demonstrated in rats, cats, fish, dogs, monkeys, and *men.* | This interference phenomenon, called learned helplessness, has been demonstrated in rats, cats, fish, dogs, monkeys, and *humans.* | Noun substituted. |
| 6. Issues raised were whether the lack of cardiac responsivity in the premature *infant* is secondary to ***his*** heightened level of autonomic arousal . . . | . . . . responsivity in the premature *infant* is secondary to ***the*** heightened level . . . | *His* changed to ***the.*** |
| | . . . . responsivity in premature *infants* is secondary to ***their*** heightened levels . . . | Rewritten in plural. |

*(continues)*

**Exhibit 4–2** continued

| Examples of common usage | Consider meaning. An alternative may be better. | Comment |
|---|---|---|
| 7. First the *individual* becomes aroused by violations of *his* personal space, and then *he* attributes the cause of this arousal to other people in *his* environment. | First *we* become aroused by violations of *our* personal space, and then *we* attribute the cause of this arousal to other people in *the* environment. | Pronouns substituted, *he* and *his* omitted. |
| 8. Much has been written about the effect that a *child's* position among *his* siblings has on *his* intellectual development. | Much has been written about the relationship between sibling position and intellectual development in *children.* | Rewritten, plural introduced. |
| 9. Subjects were 16 girls and 16 boys. Each *child* was to place a car on *his* board so that two cars and boards looked alike. | Each *child* was to place a car on *his* or *her* board so that two cars and boards looked alike. | Changed *his* to *his* or *her;* however, use sparingly to avoid monotonous repetition. *Her* or *his* may also be used, but it sounds awkward. In either case, keep pronoun order consistent to avoid ambiguity. |
| 10. Each person's alertness was measured by the difference between *his* obtained relaxation score and *his* obtained arousal score. | Each person's alertness was measured by the difference between *the* obtained relaxation and arousal scores. | *His* deleted, plural introduced. |
| 11. The client's husband *lets* her teach part-time. | The client's husband *"lets"* her teach part-time.<br><br>The husband *says* he *"lets"* the client teach part-time. | Punctuation added to clarify location of the bias, that is, with husband and wife, not with author. If necessary, rewrite to clarify as allegation. See Example 24 below. |

**Exhibit 4–2** continued

| | | |
|---|---|---|
| | The client *says her husband "lets"* her teach part-time. | |
| | B. Stereotyping | |
| 12. males, females | men, women, boys, girls, adults, children, adolescents | Specific nouns reduce possibility of stereotypic bias and often clarify discussion. Use *male* and *female* as adjectives where appropriate and relevant (female experimenter, male subject). Avoid unparallel usages such as 10 *men* and 16 *females.* |
| 13. Research scientists often neglect their *wives* and *children.* | Research scientists often neglect their *families.* | Alternative wording acknowledges that women as well as men are research scientists. |
| 14. When a *test developer* or *test user* fails to satisfy these requirements, *he* should . . . | When *test developers* or *test users* fail to satisfy these requirements, *they* should . . . | Same as Example 13. |
| 15. the psychologist . . . *he* the therapist . . . *he* the nurse . . . *she* the teacher . . . *she* | psychologists . . . *they;* the psychologist . . . *she.* therapists . . . *they;* the therapist . . . *she.* nurses . . . *they;* nurse . . . *he* teachers . . . *they;* teacher . . . he | Be specific or change to plural if discussing women as well as men. |
| 16. woman doctor, lady lawyer, male nurse | doctor, physician, lawyer, nurse | Specify sex if it is a variable or if sex designation is necessary to the discussion. ("13 female doctors and 22 male doctors"). |
| 17. mothering | parenting, nurturing (or specify exact behavior) | Noun substituted. |

*(continues)*

**Exhibit 4–2** continued

| Examples of common usage | Consider meaning. An alternative may be better. | Comment |
|---|---|---|
| 18. chairman (of an academic department) | Use *chairperson* or *chair* if it is known that the institution has established either form as an official title. Otherwise, use *chairman.* | *Department head* may be appropriate, but the term is not synonymous with *chairman* and *chairperson* at all institutions. |
| chairman (presiding officer of a committee or meeting) | chairperson, moderator, discussion leader | In parliamentary usage, *chairman* is the official term. Alternatives are acceptable in most writing. |
| 19. Only *freshmen* were eligible for the project. | (No alternative if academic standing is meant.) | *First-year student* is often an acceptable alternative to *freshman,* but in these cases, *freshmen* is used for accuracy. |
| All the students had matriculated for three years, but the majority were still *freshmen.* | | |
| 20. foreman, policeman, stewardess, mailman | supervisor, police officer, flight attendant, postal worker or letter carrier. | Noun substituted. |
| | II. Problems of Evaluation | |
| | A. Ambiguity of Referent | |
| 21. The authors acknowledge the assistance of *Mrs. John Smith.* | The authors acknowledge the assistance of *Jane Smith.* | Use given names in author acknowledgments. When forms of address are used in text, use the appropriate form: Mr., Mrs., Miss, or Ms. |
| 22. men and women, sons and daughters, boys and girls, husbands and wives | women and men, daughters and sons, girls and boys, wives and husbands | Vary the order if content does not require traditional order. |

**Exhibit 4–2** continued

| | | |
|---|---|---|
| | B. Stereotyping | |
| 23. men and girls | men and women, women and men | Use parallel terms. Of course, use *men and girls* if that is literally what is meant. |
| 24. The client's husband lets her teach part-time. | The client teaches part-time. | The author of this example intended to communicate the working status of the woman but inadvertently revealed a stereotype about husband-wife relationships; see Example 11 above. |
| 25. ambitious men and aggressive women | ambitious women and men or ambitious people<br><br>aggressive men and women or aggressive people | Some adjectives, depending on whether the person described is a man or a woman, connote bias. The examples illustrate some common usages that may not always convey exact meaning, especially when paired, as in column 1. |
| cautious men and timid women | cautious women and men, cautious people<br><br>timid men and women or timid people | |
| 26. The boys chose typically male toys. | The boys chose (specify) | Being specific reduces possibility of stereotypic bias. |
| The client's behavior was typically female. | The client's behavior was (specify) | |
| 27. woman driver | driver | If specifying sex is necessary, use *female driver.* |
| 28. The *girls* in the office greeted all clients. | secretaries, office assistants | Noun substituted. |
| 29. coed | female student | Noun substituted. |

*(continues)*

**Exhibit 4–2** continued

| Examples of common usage | Consider meaning. An alternative may be better. | Comment |
|---|---|---|
| 30. women's lib, women's libber | women's movement, feminist, supporter of women's movement | Noun substituted. |
| 31. Subjects were 16 men and 4 women. *The women were housewives.* | The men were (specify) and the women were (specify). | Describe women and men in parallel terms. *Housewife* indicates *sex,* marital status, and occupation, and excludes men. *Homemaker* indicates occupation and includes men. |

## USING ADVERTISING

Most companies and individuals who provide a product or service to the public advertise. However, most professional organizations such as The American Medical Association, The American Psychological Association, National Association for Social Workers, American Association for Marriage and Family Therapy have frowned upon advertising. Since 1977 when the Supreme Court declared that professional organizations' "ban on advertising" was in restraint of trade, a greater number of professional mental health practitioners have been experimenting with advertising.

An important caveat that should guide professionals considering advertising, whether in the mass media such as newspapers or radio or listing in the yellow pages of the phone book: *Refrain from creative advertising.* Creative advertising attempts to induce a need or a perceived need in the "eyes" of a potential user of a product or service. Advertising by professionals should be directional, that is, be an informational guide to potential consumers *when they feel a need for your services.*

### The Yellow Pages

Advertising in the yellow pages is among the most accepted and most conservative types of mental health advertising. In the past, practitioners shied away from yellow page listing because they thought it undignified, had little control over the type of person "referred," and felt that the listing was costly. Apparently this is not the case today. In 1961 when I arrived in Rochester, New York, clutching my newly obtained Ph.D., there were only a few psychologists, six, who listed their services in the yellow pages, with none of the six engaged in full-time private practice. In 1980 there were 48 psychologists advertising in the yellow pages, with at least ten practicing independently on a full-time basis.

The National Resource Center for Consumer and Legal Services, Inc., reported that in 1980 for every dollar spent on advertising, attorneys received an average of 7.93 dollars in fees. The yellow pages can provide directional type information to clients already in need of your services. Such information as location, office hours, and specialization, for example, is what they would require. Furthermore, the yellow pages can provide the same information to possible referral sources who may want to refer to a mental health specialist in their own town or village rather than use the clinician who may be based at the medical center many miles away.

Advertising in the yellow pages is visual. Having your listing stand apart from your colleagues can be helpful and will not violate professional ethics. Bold type, a box, listing of specialty or ABPP status can draw potential clients' attention to your listing.

**Community Talks**

Talking in the community is a tried and true method of informing referral sources such as teachers, guidance counselors, clergy, as well as possible patients, about yourself. Especially if you are new to the community, giving talks can help get you established quickly. A brief note identifying your credentials and the listing of some topics you feel qualified to talk on usually gets results. Exhibit 4–3 presents an example of such a letter. Chapter 7 will provide details, the "nuts and bolts" of making the actual presentations.

Once a date is arrived at you can inquire whether the group has a publicity chairperson or if not, as is usually the case, whether there would be any objection to your sending a news release to the local newspapers announcing the talk.

Local school, church, or temple groups are often interested in sponsoring a series of related talks or miniworkshops. Many people who attend such "courses" need psychotherapy and between 5 and 10 percent usually wind up seeking therapy. The investment of time generally turns out to be a good one.

**Newspapers**

News items, interviews, and feature stories that center around you and your work can be stimulating and productive. A feature article on a psychologist specializing in career planning and vocational evaluation began: "I wouldn't hire anybody based only on a resume." The clear implication of the

**Exhibit 4–3** Sample Letter for Speaking Functions

Stanley Kissel, Ph.D.
1425 Portland Avenue
Rochester, New York 14620

Dear

I am writing to inform you that I am now available to speak with parents and educators on a number of topics relating to children and youth, their development and their problems.

I have been affiliated with the Children and Youth Division of the Rochester Medical Center and am also in private practice.

I would be most interested in talking on the following topics:

..... Hyperactivity and Learning Disabilities
..... The Effects of Divorce on Children
..... Childhood Depression
..... Communicating with Adolescents

I look forward to working with your group.

Sincerely yours,

Stanley Kissel, Ph.D.
Diplomate American Board
of Professional Psychologists,
Inc.

article, which was quite informative, suggested that psychological services were a helpful and necessary part of an executive hiring package. Were such a provocative statement part of a paid advertisement it would raise many eyebrows in the professional community.

The following "checklist" is based on the standard for public information and advertising (Psychotherapy Finances Guide to Private Practice, 1980).

• *What marriage counselors can put in ads*—In an effort to come to terms with new realities of professional advertising, the American Association for Marriage and Family Therapy recently issued its set of standards for public information in advertising. Rather than try to tell members what they can do, it goes into great detail on what to avoid, dotting more i's and crossing more t's than ethics codes of other societies. While there is still a great deal of ground for interpretation, many of the "don'ts" are a useful checklist for all therapists considering advertising.

• *Self-praising should be avoided,* not only in the actual statements made but also in volume, scope, or frequency of ads, or by use of unrepresentative biographical information. Use of an inappropriate media can be self praising.
• *Fee information demands special care* since it is difficult to make it really complete or accurate enough to avoid deceiving a lay person. Of course, if a set fee is advertised for a specific type of case, it should be adhered to.
• *Past performance results are tricky,* as is other information that is advertised without explaining all-important variables—often impossible to do in ads.
• *Only facts, not opinions, should be stated*—These should not only be truthful but their accurate meanings should be apparent to the average lay person.
• *No guarantees about the outcomes of therapy* should be made or even implied.
• *Watch out for appeals to fear* in seeking business, or the use of brash or extravagant statements, since these could mislead or harm the lay person.
• *Don't use misleading names* that could give an erroneous impression about your identity, responsibility, or status, or improperly implied links to any group.

Advertising by professionals is a new venture. There has been more concern with creating false hopes in the minds of the public or taking an unprofessional posture. Those who are interested in advertising would do well to consider the following two "dos."

- Emphasize your specialty by aiming at a particular type of client, such as a single parent, senior citizen, the recently widowed, etc. Ads can be a way to get to specific types of potential patients you want to reach without waiting for word of mouth.
- Mention your expertise, especially if you recently completed specialized training or have special therapy skills that you know are needed in your community.

Advertising is a way of helping you get established quickly in a new area, especially if it's a city or town that's loaded with clinicians. Of course, you're risking the possibility of alienating potential referral sources, but in a highly competitive situation you might not really have a chance to build a practice through traditional referrals.

Although somewhat more controversial, it is neither unethical nor unprofessional to include an appropriate presentation of fee information in an advertisement. Exhibit 4–4 is an example of an announcement-advertisement that incorporates some of the points we have been making.

**Exhibit 4–4** Sample Announcement-Advertisement

STANLEY KISSEL, PH. D.
announces the opening of his office for the general practice of clinical psychology.
I am particularly interested in providing consultation, evaluation, and treatment services to learning disabled children and their families.
Saturday and evening hours. 123 Street, Rochester, New York 14600 123-5678.

## Public Service Messages

A somewhat more "daring" approach to advertising is the public service message. This can be helpful for an established practitioner who feels the practice may need a "bolster shot." What is involved is offering your services to local newspapers, radio, or TV on a quid pro quo basis, exchanging your time for their exposure. However, while most newspapers feature columns that answer questions of their readers or express opinions, unless you have a national reputation, they are unlikely to furnish you a forum to show your wares to the public.

Dentists, family practice physicians, and other professionals have been experimenting with the paid-for public service column. This, too, is something ycu might want to consider. An example that is relevant to the practice of mental health is presented in Exhibit 4–5.

## SUMMARY

The marketing strategies that have been presented in this chapter are costly both in terms of time and money. They are meant to bring your name before the community for possible referral sources and clients. Of course, they are not a substitute for a good reputation or personal acquaintances. In the next chapter we will consider some marketing strategies that are especially relevant to the mental health practitioner who is considering establishing a part-time practice while working for a public agency, or who is already in part-time practice and wants an expanded referral base.

**Exhibit 4–5** A Sample Advertising Column

# VIEWS ON MENTAL HEALTH

**by Stanley Kissel, Ph.D.**

## FACTS ABOUT MENTAL HEALTH

Emotional problems, unlike certain physical ailments, may take many years to develop to the point where symptoms cause concern and worry to the individual. The symptoms are indicators of too-heavy burdens, stresses and conflicts. What are some of these signs for children? Mental health experts agree that the following are possible danger signals:

..Prolonged periods of unhappiness without apparent cause.

..Refusal to accept school or parental authority.

..Persistent avoidance of school.

..Excessive fears which are upsetting and interfere with normal function.

..Poor achievement in school subjects.

..Returning to activities associated with infancy, such as frequent (not occasional) bedwetting, soiling, head-banging, thumb sucking, and little ability to tolerate frustration.

If too many of these signals are present, a consultation with your family physician, clergyman, school counselor or a mental health expert may be helpful. . . .

*A public service with the aim of promoting a better mental health environment from the offices of Mid-State Psychological Services, 1420 Axle Street, Rochester, New York. Phone: 123-4567*

Chapter 5

# Marketing That Can Make a Difference

# 5

Although full-time private practice is looked upon as an attractive option for mental health specialists, the majority of clinicians are initially employed by public health care agencies. A recent survey of the American Psychological Association revealed that 35 percent of new Ph.D. graduates are employed by such health care agencies as hospitals, clinics, and community mental health centers, whereas 3 percent are independent private practitioners (Dorken & Webb, 1980).

The practitioner who is in public practice can use the public platform offered by the clinic, mental health center, hospital, or university to the betterment of both public and private professional identity. He or she comes in contact with a number of possible referral sources, i.e., internists, guidance counselors, parole officers, youth workers, school principals, lawyers, and pediatricians in the course of agency conferences. The type of reports provided to referral sources becomes another way of identifying yourself and provides the opportunity to build up a personal following of referral sources. Clients referred to your agency begin to see you as *their* service provider. Some public agencies try to comply with such requests, others do not consider themselves a "consortium of private practitioners." Ultimately, the referral source will begin to develop a relationship with you and, where appropriate, will refer to you as an independent practitioner.

Two innovative techniques, teaching assessments and linking, are procedures that alloy good clinical practice with wise marketing and ultimately benefit all—practitioner, client, and referral source. These two approaches will be the focus of this chapter.

## TEACHING ASSESSMENTS

Teaching assessments are diagnostic and evaluative workups that result in educationally oriented reports, conferences, and feedback. The referring professional gets educated as well as having the referral questions answered. This gives you the opportunity to "toot your own horn" while providing a great deal of information about the client who is being evaluated. Although it is somewhat more practical to provide teaching-oriented assessments at case conferences, they can be done in a written report.

There are four components in this type of assessment package:

1. A description of the test instrument, or the techniques used to generate your conclusions.
2. The normal expectations or responses of the test.
3. The client's reactions and responses.
4. Expectations or responses of individuals having related problems. When appropriate, indicate differential diagnosis.

For example, when attending a school conference with teaching staff, principal, and guidance counselors where the concern centers around learning disability, I would describe the *Wechsler Intelligence Scale for Children-Revised,* typical reactions of normal children and those who have difficulty with learning but for different reasons, and then the conferenced child's response to the test.

A report of a nine-year-old child referred because of reading difficulty will be used to illustrate a practical application of a teaching assessment conference. Although a complete battery of psychological and psychoeducational tests was administered, we will concern ourselves only with the WISC-R.

Bobby, a third-grader, was having continued difficulty in comprehension skills but was able to decode at grade level. Medical examinations revealed normal vision and hearing. The following WISC-R profile was obtained:

| | |
|---|---|
| Verbal subtest scaled scores: | |
| Information | 7 |
| Comprehension | 5 |
| Similarities | 6 |
| Vocabulary | 12 |
| Digit Span | 12 |
| Performance subtest scaled scores: | |
| Picture Completion | 15 |
| Picture Arrangement | 14 |

| | |
|---|---|
| Block Design | 8 |
| Object Assembly | 12 |
| Coding | 9 |
| Verbal IQ | 97 |
| Performance IQ | 111 |
| Full Scale IQ | 103 |
| Verbal scaled scores | 9.5 |
| Performance scaled score | 11.6 |

## Description of Diagnostic Procedures

The first step at the conference was to focus the attention to the referral problems, i.e., the boy's limited ability to read, reflecting possible intellectual limitations or psychoeducational deficiencies.

The next step was to introduce and describe in detail the test(s) chosen. The WISC-R, an individually administered intelligence test, was selected because it is the most reliable and valid objective measure of intelligence and in addition to providing a measure of intellectual functioning, it provides information regarding:

- the ability to understand and solve problems
- the ability to retain knowledge
- the ability to reason
- the child's predominant mode of learning

A blank WISC-R profile form was shown (see Exhibit 5–1) and each subtest described.

The WISC-R consists of two sections, a verbal scale and a performance scale, each having five required subtests and one alternate. The subtests are administered alternatively to maximize a child's interest and motivational level. Excessive frustration is minimized for a child who is deficient in either verbal or performance skills. The questions of the various subtests are presented in an ascending order, going from easy to more difficult.

**Exhibit 5–1** WISC-R Record Form

# WISC-R RECORD FORM

**Wechsler Intelligence Scale for Children—Revised**

NAME ______ AGE ____ SEX ____

ADDRESS ______

PARENT'S NAME ______

SCHOOL ______ GRADE ______

PLACE OF TESTING ______ TESTED BY ______

REFERRED BY ______

## WISC-R PROFILE

Clinicians who wish to draw a profile should first transfer the child's *scaled* scores to the row of boxes below. Then mark an X on the dot corresponding to the scaled score for each test, and draw a line connecting the X's.*

| | VERBAL TESTS | | | | | | | PERFORMANCE TESTS | | | | | | |
|---|---|---|---|---|---|---|---|---|---|---|---|---|---|---|
| Scaled Score | Information | Similarities | Arithmetic | Vocabulary | Comprehension | Digit Span | Scaled Score | Picture Completion | Picture Arrangement | Block Design | Object Assembly | Coding | Mazes | Scaled Score |
| | ☐ | ☐ | ☐ | ☐ | ☐ | ☐ | | ☐ | ☐ | ☐ | ☐ | ☐ | ☐ | |
| 19 | • | • | • | • | • | • | 19 | • | • | • | • | • | • | 19 |
| 18 | • | • | • | • | • | • | 18 | • | • | • | • | • | • | 18 |
| 17 | • | • | • | • | • | • | 17 | • | • | • | • | • | • | 17 |
| 16 | • | • | • | • | • | • | 16 | • | • | • | • | • | • | 16 |
| 15 | • | • | • | • | • | • | 15 | • | • | • | • | • | • | 15 |
| 14 | • | • | • | • | • | • | 14 | • | • | • | • | • | • | 14 |
| 13 | • | • | • | • | • | • | 13 | • | • | • | • | • | • | 13 |
| 12 | • | • | • | • | • | • | 12 | • | • | • | • | • | • | 12 |
| 11 | • | • | • | • | • | • | 11 | • | • | • | • | • | • | 11 |
| 10 | • | • | • | • | • | • | 10 | • | • | • | • | • | • | 10 |
| 9 | • | • | • | • | • | • | 9 | • | • | • | • | • | • | 9 |
| 8 | • | • | • | • | • | • | 8 | • | • | • | • | • | • | 8 |
| 7 | • | • | • | • | • | • | 7 | • | • | • | • | • | • | 7 |
| 6 | • | • | • | • | • | • | 6 | • | • | • | • | • | • | 6 |
| 5 | • | • | • | • | • | • | 5 | • | • | • | • | • | • | 5 |
| 4 | • | • | • | • | • | • | 4 | • | • | • | • | • | • | 4 |
| 3 | • | • | • | • | • | • | 3 | • | • | • | • | • | • | 3 |
| 2 | • | • | • | • | • | • | 2 | • | • | • | • | • | • | 2 |
| 1 | • | • | • | • | • | • | 1 | • | • | • | • | • | • | 1 |

*See Chapter 4 in the manual for a discussion of the significance of differences between scores on the tests.

| | Year | Month | Day |
|---|---|---|---|
| Date Tested | ____ | ____ | ____ |
| Date of Birth | ____ | ____ | ____ |
| Age | ____ | ____ | ____ |

| | Raw Score | Scaled Score |
|---|---|---|
| **VERBAL TESTS** | | |
| Information | ____ | ____ |
| Similarities | ____ | ____ |
| Arithmetic | ____ | ____ |
| Vocabulary | ____ | ____ |
| Comprehension | ____ | ____ |
| (Digit Span) | (____) | (____) |
| Verbal Score | | ____ |
| **PERFORMANCE TESTS** | | |
| Picture Completion | ____ | ____ |
| Picture Arrangement | ____ | ____ |
| Block Design | ____ | ____ |
| Object Assembly | ____ | ____ |
| Coding | ____ | ____ |
| (Mazes) | (____) | (____) |
| Performance Score | | ____ |

| | Scaled Score | IQ |
|---|---|---|
| Verbal Score | ____* | ____ |
| Performance Score | ____* | ____ |
| Full Scale Score | ____ | ____ |

*Prorated from 4 tests, if necessary.

NOTES

*Verbal Subtests*

• *Information*—30 questions covering a wide variety of general information. The questions are factual, requiring very brief answers. The child is not required to find relationships between facts but has only to demonstrate that these facts have been stored as general knowledge. Therefore, this test measures a learned fund of knowledge gained from experience and education. The following questions are examples that are similar but not identical to questions in the WISC-R information subtests:

"How many eyes do you have?"

"What is the last month of the year?"

"How many minutes are there in an hour?"

• *Comprehension*—17 items designed to discover social judgment and practical common sense in reasoning. The subtest is not a measure of *reading comprehension.* Examples of similar but not identical items are:

"What are some reasons we need firemen?"

"What is the thing to do if you find something that you like but it belongs to one of your friends?"

• *Arithmetic*—15 arithmetic problems are presented orally. The child is required to do these mental computations without paper or pencil during a specific time period. Three problems are presented visually to be read by the child. In addition to measuring arithmetic skills, this test provides information on a child's ability to concentrate, attend, and remember. The questions are similar to those encountered in elementary arithmetic.

• *Similarities*—17 items that require the child to say how items are similar. For example: "How are coal and gasoline alike?" The test measures abstract thinking and verbal concept formation.

• *Vocabulary*—asks a child to define words presented both visually and orally. The vocabulary subtest is considered to be the best single verbal measure of general intelligence on the WISC-R. It provides information regarding a child's word knowledge, richness of ideas, and proficiency of verbal expression.

• *Digit Span*—two parts: on the first part the child is asked to repeat a series of digits and on the second part to repeat a different series of digits backwards. This test provides information on auditory sequential memory, concentration, and attention.

*Performance Subtests*

• *Picture Completion*—26 pictures, each containing an important missing part to be identified. This is a timed test. Picture completion measures a child's sensitivity to detail and visual perception.

• *Picture Arrangement*—each task consists of a number of picture cards presented in a scrambled order. In a fixed time period, they must be arranged sequentially so they tell a meaningful story. The subtest measures visual perception, attention to detail, visual sequencing, and cause-effect relationships.

• *Block Design*—child is required to reproduce picture designs with colored blocks within a specified time period. The subtest measures nonverbal abstract problem solving, analytic thinking, and spatial relationships. The block design subtest is the best single measure of nonverbal intelligence on the WISC-R.

• *Object Assembly*—four separate noninterlocking puzzle-like objects that must be combined to make up a familiar object. Success on this task is more dependent on visualizing the whole rather than on the shape of the pieces. This is a timed test that measures visual-motor ability, visual integration, and part-whole relationships. The child uses inductive reasoning (working toward the whole from parts without a model).

• *Coding*—child is presented a code of symbols that match a series of numbers. Exhibit 5–2 presents a facsimile of the coding task. The child is shown the code and then has to fill in as many of the 93 blanks that he or she can in a two-minute period. This subtest measures speed and accuracy of visual-motor ability as well as visual memory.

When the WISC-R was created, a standard score of 100 was set as average, with most normal children falling within 15 points (85 to 115). Although children will show some variability from one subtest to another and between overall verbal and performance ability, subscale scatter of three or more points and verbal-performance discrepancies of 15 or more points are considered significant. Children who are mentally retarded usually show minimal verbal-performance discrepancies, with their overall performance falling below 69; whereas normal children of average or above average intelligence also show insignificant scatter but their overall functioning is 90 or above.

In the next phase of the conference the clinician brings the focus back to the child who was referred for study. Now let's consider Bobby's response to the WISC-R.

The Full Scale IQ of 103 places Bobby within the average range of intellectual functioning. The 14-point differential between the verbal and performance IQ scores suggests that the child's general strengths are in the performance area, which is typically found in children with reading disabilities. Bobby's performance IQ is 111 and places him in the bright normal range of intelligence, which indicates that his current level of functioning is

**Exhibit 5–2** The Coding Subtest: A Facsimile

| 1 | 2 | 3 | 4 | 5 |
|---|---|---|---|---|
| O | X | — | N | < |

| 1 | 5 | 3 | 2 | 1 | 5 | 4 | 3 | 2 | 5 | 1 | 4 |
|---|---|---|---|---|---|---|---|---|---|---|---|
| | | | | | | | | | | | |

an underestimation of his ability. It is clear that Bobby has difficulty receiving and processing information presented auditorially but does well with nonverbal processes.

An analysis of the subtest scores reveals that arithmetic, block design, and similarities deviate significantly from his own standard score. Information and coding are also low but not significantly.

These low areas indicate a child who is still at a concrete stage of development and has difficulty conceptualizing and thinking abstractly. Without these skills, reading comprehension will be hindered greatly. Significant strengths are found in comprehension, vocabulary, picture completion, and picture arrangement. The child has a sophisticated vocabulary.

These high scores suggest that Bobby's environment has been enriching, allowing him to have good social judgment, word knowledge, and sensitivity to details in his visual environment.

### Recommendation

Since Bobby is unable to understand reading material through content alone, a reading series that is highly graphic should be used. Two-dimensional pictures should help him understand what the words are saying. Reading material should be at a simple level in content matter even though he can decode at grade level and has a sophisticated vocabulary.

Comprehension questions should be presented before Bobby reads the material, in addition to his reading. This will cue him into reading for comprehension. Teaching of new words should depend upon linguistic skills and sight vocabulary repetition rather than the use of content. The cloze technique, a remedial procedure that omits selected words from the story, will help in strengthening comprehension skills.

If additional tests were administered, the same procedure would be repeated so that after discussing the WISC-R and Bobby's performance on the test, I would then introduce the next test before discussing my conclusions and recommendations. For example, if the Bender-Gestalt Visual-Motor Test was also administered, I would describe that test. The Bender-Gestalt requires a child to copy a series of nine geometric designs. The degree to which the designs can be accurately copied gives a measure of visual-motor integration skills that relate to brain damage in adults and perceptual development in children. The size of figures copied, placement of the drawings, and execution of the task provide information about emotional reactivity.

Specific signs have been identified reflecting typical Bender-Gestalt errors in children with brain dysfunction and emotional disturbance but it is hazardous to make such inferences before age eight or nine. By age ten perceptual motor maturation has reached a point where analysis of copying errors can often differentiate between organic and emotional problems.

A number of errors indicating gross misperception of shapes, inability to make complex designs, seeing angles for curves, and clear rotation of designs are more typically associated with cerebral dysfunction; errors such as overestimation or underestimation of size, heavy reworking of lines, and confused order of copying are more typically associated with emotional problems. When a child produces both kinds of signs it can usually be inferred that the child is having some emotional problems in adjusting to perceptual-motor difficulties.

If personality tests were administered I would discuss them next. I would first make some general comments about projective techniques and then give a brief description of the ones administered.

Projective techniques provide the opportunity for the expression of personality dimensions in a semistructured situation. Information on such personality traits as aggression, need for achievement, dependency, power, anxiety, frustration, tolerance, and emotional maturity are obtained on such projective techniques as the Rorschach, Draw-a-Person, and the Thematic Apperception Test. The Rorschach consists of ten ink blots of various shades of black, gray, red, and pastel colors that are presented one at a time with instructions to "Tell me what it looks like or what it might be." Everything else is left to the subject: how many things seen (number of responses), what part of the ink blot used (location), what features of the ink blot used (determinant), what kind of things seen (content), and type of communication (verbalization). The characteristics of the responses—location, use of determinants, content preferences, and style of verbalization—provide the data on which Rorschach interpretations are based.

In the Thematic Apperception Test (TAT) or Children's Apperception Test (CAT) the patient is shown a series of pictures and asked to create a story about each one with a beginning, middle, and ending. The TAT pictures involve people, whereas in the CAT animals are used in order to facilitate the responsiveness of younger children.

The time constraints, the number of techniques administered, the level of sophistication of the conferees will, of course, determine the depth and elaborateness of your presentation.

## FEEDBACK REPORTS

Although face-to-face conferences provide the optimal format for teaching-oriented feedback, they are costly and time consuming. More often clinicians, whether public or private, full time or part time, feed back information briefly on the telephone or via reports. Let us now consider the written feedback report as a vehicle for teaching-oriented evaluations. The following basic information should be included in a feedback report to a referral source:

- *Referral and Client Information*
  1. Name
  2. Date of birth
  3. Referral source
  4. Referral question
- *Background*
  1. Educational/vocational history
  2. Developmental history of child
  3. Important family losses (separations, divorces, deaths, hospitalizations)
  4. Peer relationships
  5. Physical health status
- *Techniques—Tests administered*

List all tests if a traditional report. Describe in detail some or all tests if a teaching-oriented report.

- *Behavior during evaluation*
  1. Patient-diagnostic interactions (hostile, resistant, timid, cooperative, outgoing)

2. Affect (anxious, depressed)
3. Attention span (focused, distractible)
4. Reactions to frustration (anxious, sullen, withdrawn, persistent)
5. General behavior (unusual behaviors, strange or inappropriate verbalization, blocking)

- *Intellectual Evaluation* (if appropriate)
  1. Current level of intellectual functioning
  2. Estimate of intellectual potential
  3. Configuration of intellectual strengths and weaknesses

The form shown in Exhibit 5–3 is one way of including the information in teaching-oriented reports.

- *Emotional Functioning*
  1. Self-concept
  2. Interpersonal perceptions and actions
  3. Major defense mechanism
  4. Level of emotional maturity
  5. Situational aspects of emotional reactivity, i.e., need for structure, or ability to function with minimal directions
- *Diagnosis* (optional but helpful and often necessary for insurance purposes). The *Diagnostic and Statistical Manual III,* published by American Psychiatric Association, is helpful for designating a diagnosis.
- *Recommendations*
  1. Environmental change, i.e., home, school, or work
  2. Personality change, i.e., psychotherapy, behavior modification, or medication
  3. Concrete suggestions for implementing your recommendations whenever possible.

## A Sample Case

The following example is one way of integrating a teaching-oriented feedback report with a more traditionally oriented report.

Margaret, a 13½-year-old seventh-grader whose physical appearance is consistent with her chronological age, was referred by the school social worker because of poor school adjustment. During the past three years Margaret has been in a learning disabilities class for children thought to be of average intelligence but unable to achieve. She repeated second grade and was found to be reading at a mid-first-grade level at the end of third grade. At that time an intellectual evaluation found her to be functioning in the borderline range

**Exhibit 5–3** Intelligence Summary Form

WECHSLER INTELLIGENCE SCALES PROFILE FORM

________WAIS ________WISC-R ________WPPSI

Scaled scores can range between 1-19. Those between 8-12 fall within the normal range.

TEST FINDINGS: Verbal Scale IQ ________
Performance Scale IQ ________
Full Scale IQ ________

| Verbal Scale Subtests | Scaled Score | Performance Scale Subtests | Scaled Score |
|---|---|---|---|
| *Information*<br>Information gained from experience educational, intellectual effort, alertness to world around, memory retention. | ________ | *Picture Completion*<br>Visual alertness and organization, ability to recognize essential details, contact with reality, requires attention. | ________ |
| *Comprehension*<br>Practical knowledge and social judgment, anticipation and judging consequences, (poor verbalizers often score low), reasoning ability. | ________ | *Picture Arrangement*<br>Nonverbal judgment, anticipation, and planning (through use of essential pictured clues), responsiveness to interpersonal relationships, good foresight. | ________ |
| *Arithmetic*<br>Concentration and arithmetic reasoning, specific school learning, mental alertness. | ________ | *Block Design*<br>Best single nonlanguage test, analysis and reproduction of abstract designs, logical insight into space relationships, visual motor perception coordination. | ________ |
| *Similarities*<br>Ability to recognize and describe essential relations between objects or ideas, i.e., verbal concept information, concrete vs. abstract kinds of thinking. | ________ | *Object Assembly*<br>Seeing relationships of parts to the whole in a familiar configuration, carefulness and persistence at a task, critical appraisal of small details. | ________ |
| *Vocabulary*<br>Best single measure of verbal intelligence and learning ability, cultural environment reflected, potentiality for dealing with symbols, quality and character of thought process. | ________ | *Coding Digit Symbol*<br>Speed of motor-visual reaction and association of symbols, ability to learn an unfamiliar task (low coding indicates poor visual motor coordination). | ________ |

*(continues)*

**Exhibit 5–3** continued

| Verbal Scale Subtests | Scaled Score | Performance Scale Subtests | Scaled Score |
|---|---|---|---|
| | *ALTERNATE TESTS* | | |
| *Digit Span*<br>Attention and auditory memory, self-control (low score indicates tension), measures anxiety. | ______ | *Mazes*<br>Foresight, planning, and following a visual pattern. | ______ |

of intelligence (WISC-R Verbal IQ 70, Performance IQ 89, Full Scale IQ 77). The estimate was considered to be a minimal one. She also had difficulty accurately copying the Bender-Gestalt designs—distorting their shapes—and was reported to show strange behaviors in class.

Margaret's parents obtained a divorce four years ago. She, a younger, and older sister remained with her mother while an older mentally retarded child went to live with father. The maternal grandmother as well as mother's half brother were also believed to be mentally retarded. Margaret's developmental history was uneventful except for the fact that she walked at 16 months and was a head banger. During 1971–72 she was in psychotherapy due to withdrawn behavior. Therapy was terminated at the end of that school year as she improved, although Margaret was thought to be a "child at risk."

At the present time her teacher reports her to be resistant in the classroom, refusing to turn in homework or complete assignments and finding it extremely difficult to get along with the other children. The teachers question whether or not Margaret is appropriately placed.

Margaret was seen for psychological evaluation on February 3, and administered the following tests: WISC-R, Rorschach, TAT, Draw-a-Person, Bender-Gestalt, and WRAT (reading section).

Margaret, a dark-complexioned girl, was glancing at a magazine and subtly rocking in the waiting room. She became perceptibly more anxious when introduced to me, which caused her to distort her facial features and make a dull look in appearance. She slowly accompanied me to the testing room, clutching at her coat, which she wore for the entire two-hour testing session. Margaret found it difficult to talk with me regarding the purpose of our meeting but agreed she was not pleased with school. She spoke in a soft, hesitant fashion, at times mispronouncing words, which further contributed to the impression of dullness. Although eye contact was good, attempts to get Margaret to elaborate on ambiguous, vague responses were often met with "I can't" or an abrupt turning away. When asked to justify a discrepancy between her drawings of one of the Bender-Gestalt designs she commented, "I didn't feel like making more dots."

After about a half hour Margaret was able to relax, smile, laugh appropriately, and her facial features softened, suggesting that with better grooming she could be an attractive young lady.

At the conclusion of our session Margaret showed less hesitancy in talking and informed me she did not want to return to school but would rather stay home with her mother. If she had to attend, then she wished to be placed in a different class. Margaret complained that the children tease her about her appearance. Softly she commented, "I wish I was more like the other kids."

Currently Margaret is functioning within the retarded range of intelligence (Verbal IQ 65, Performance IQ 63, Full Scale IQ 60). As can be seen from the WISC-R profile chart in Exhibit 5–4 her performance on a wide variety of cognitive tasks varies from the borderline to the severely retarded. She had most difficulty when asked to demonstrate school-related skills such as a fund of general information, computational skills, or social awareness. This is not surprising in light of her history of chronic school failure and her current reading level, which is at the second grade. Margaret showed relatively better ability to concentrate and attend to a series of familiar objects that had some meaning for her. On other tasks that required similar skills, such as remembering a series of numbers or learning meaningless symbols, she found it more difficult to concentrate. Comparing her current level of intellectual functioning with previous functioning suggests that Margaret is decompensating. However, her achievement level has remained relatively constant (WRAT reading score 1.6; arithmetic K-7) over the past three years; furthermore, visual-motor and personality tests did not suggest the presence of regression or overwhelming anxiety that would cause extreme inefficiencies in intellectual functioning.

Margaret's achievements on the Bender-Gestalt Visual-Motor Test were at the eight-year level. She was asked to copy nine geometric designs without any time limit. By the age of ten most normal children are able to copy the designs with good accuracy and commit less than two errors. Margaret made five errors, most of which involved simplification. Gross distortion and perseveration errors were not present. These errors are often found in individuals who show severe emotional disabilities.

Margaret, however, does show a low self-concept and has significant emotional disturbance. Although she has limited ability, she seems to exaggerate her limitations in the sense that she quickly gives up in the face of mild frustration and is easily hurt.

Emotional immaturity was strikingly evident throughout the record. Her drawing was poorly proportioned, more childlike than adolescent. She was unable to perceive humans on the Rorschach and seemed more involved in

**Exhibit 5–4** Wechsler Intelligence Scales Profile Form

WECHSLER INTELLIGENCE SCALES PROFILE FORM

_______ WAIS ___X___ WISC-R _______ WPPSI

Scaled scores can range between 1–19. Those between 8–12 fall within the normal range.

TEST FINDINGS:

| | | |
|---|---|---|
| TEST FINDINGS: | Verbal Scale IQ | 65 |
| | Performance Scale IQ | 63 |
| | Full Scale IQ | 60 |

| Verbal Scale Subtests | Scaled Score |
|---|---|
| *Information* — Information gained from experience educational, intellectual effort, alertness to world around him, memory retention. | 4 |
| *Comprehension* — Practical knowledge and social judgement, anticipation and judging consequences, (poor verbalizers often score low), reasoning ability. | 4 |
| *Arithmetic* — Concentration and arithmetic reasoning, specific school learning, mental alertness. | 3 |
| *Similarities* — Ability to recognize and describe essential relations between objects or ideas, i.e., verbal concept information, concrete vs. abstract kinds of thinking. | 6 |
| *Vocabulary* — Best single measure of verbal intelligence and learning ability, cultural environment reflected, potentiality for dealing with symbols, quality and character of thought process. | 4 |

| Performance Scale Subtests | Scaled Score |
|---|---|
| *Picture Completion* — Visual alertness and organization, ability to recognize essential details, contact with reality, requires attention. good visual organization. | 7 |
| *Picture Arrangement* — Nonverbal judgement, anticipation, and planning (through use of essential pictured clues); responsiveness to interpersonal relationships, good foresight. | 4 |
| *Block Design* — Best single nonlanguage test, analysis and reproduction of abstract designs, logical insight into space relationships, visual motor perception coordination. | 4 |
| *Object Assembly* — Seeing relationships of parts to the whole in a familiar configuration, carefulness and persistence at a task, critical appraisal of small details. | 4 |
| *Coding Digit Symbol* — Speed of motor-visual reaction and association of symbols, ability to learn an unfamiliar task (low coding indicates poor visual motor coordination). | 3 |

**Exhibit 5–4** continued

*ALTERNATE TESTS*

| | | | |
|---|---|---|---|
| *Digit Span*<br>Attention and auditory memory; self-control (low score indicates tension), measures anxiety. | 4 | *Mazes*<br>Foresight, planning, and following a visual pattern. | ______ |

child-parent relationship problems than in peer-oriented ones. Feelings of helplessness and a surface need to avoid experiencing hostility toward maternal figures make it difficult for Margaret to come to grips with her limitations. This will be a barrier toward the development of more self-reliant skills. Emotional immaturity was most striking on the least structured tasks, such as the Draw-a-Person and Rorschach. While Margaret looks to fantasy for gratification and sees the external environment as frustrating and threatening, she has not retreated to a world of fantasy, nor are her perceptions so arbitrary as to distort reality. Impulsivity, inability to anticipate the consequences of her actions, and an inability to reflect on her behavior make Margaret seem more disorganized, chaotic, and less capable than she is.

Denial and avoidance of action are among the major psychological defenses that Margaret uses to handle anxiety. While they are relatively effective in helping her tolerate feelings of discomfort, they have hindered her interpersonal and intellectual development.

On the positive side is Margaret's wish to relate to people and her willingness and ability to form interpersonal relationships. That she was able to benefit from psychotherapy in the past and show some change in her behavior during the testing session are two indications that Margaret has the capacity to benefit from human relationships when she feels accepted in nonthreatening situations.

In summary, Margaret is a mentally retarded girl who has made little school progress during the last three years. Some of her current troublesome school behavior can be understood as a reaction to a new school. But for the most part her intellectual-emotional limitations and immaturity make it difficult for her to shift from parent-oriented relationships to peer-oriented ones with their associated "give and take." She longs for the security of her home where she can feel protected by her mother. It is recommended that Margaret be placed in a class for the mentally retarded with a teacher who can provide nurturance and sympathetic understanding. The teacher should encourage Margaret to use her abilities to solve tasks that are within her grasp.

Since Margaret performs poorly in group situations, individualized tutoring to develop practical and essential arithmetic skills, such as handling money, is needed. Margaret should be provided opportunities to associate with schoolmates of her own chronological age. Mainstreaming her in such classes as gym, art, and music would provide this opportunity. It is also suggested that Margaret return to psychotherapy so that she may derive maximum benefits from her school program and gain help in coming to grips with her limitations.

### Cover Sheet

When sending out reports, especially to schools, or agencies where many people have access to the information, it is wise to attach a cover sheet that includes the following points:

> This evaluation is a confidential interpretation regarding the abilities, aptitudes, and personality characteristics of [name of client]. Treat the material in a confidential manner, share it only with those who will be working with [name of client], and do not reproduce any portion of the report.
>
> The material contained in this evaluation may become invalid over time, so bear in mind the date of the report.

## LINKING

The very effective marketing procedure called linking emerged from working with community public human service providers.

A survey was conducted of 52 pediatricians in 32 private practices to determine their impressions of psychiatric consultation with a community child guidance clinic. Their comments were correlated with data from clinic records over a five-year-period. Prolonged waiting for initial service and ineffective communication were major problems voiced by pediatricians and confirmed by clinic records (Thorpe & Halpern, 1965).

Improvements in these problems can occur when attention is given to more expeditious intake procedures, to a better use of professional coordination, and to improved educational programs in mental health care (Thorpe & Halpern, 1965). On cases that I was asked to evaluate, I began feeding back information rapidly by phone and followed that up with written teaching-oriented reports. One group of three pediatricians, all of whom were mental health oriented, invited me to discuss an affiliative relationship. Two meetings were held in order to familiarize me with what it would be like seeing patients within the confines of a pediatric office. This also provided an opportunity for the pediatricians and me to develop a closer working relationship. Such details as the procedures for referrals, the scheduling of appointments, the rental of office space, the nature of the billing procedures, as well as how to introduce me to the pediatric patient pool were discussed. My name was placed on the door of the office, a consultation room was provided, and I made myself available to the group for four hours a week. A quid pro quo was worked out: mainly, the pediatricians were able to provide quick psychological service for their patients and I had a reliable referral source in a rent-free office. This arrangement was worked out over fifteen years ago and is still going strong.

At the suggestion of local school personnel referrals for psychological consultation were patient initiated. Peculiar physical or social mannerisms displayed by the child during a routine physical examination was another reason for referrals. The initial appointment was arranged by the pediatrician's receptionist (to promote a feeling of continuity of service) for the child's parents to meet with me. Although much of the information the parents discussed during the session (developmental data, family history, the child's symptoms) was available, this meeting afforded me the chance to get an independent impression of the family, especially the "family milieu." It also gave the parent an opportunity to raise questions regarding the psychological consultation, as well as to discuss preparation of the child. Thus a working relationship between the child's parents and myself was initiated at the first visit. Two or three sessions with the child followed. The service culminated in a parent conference where the family experiences were reviewed and initial concerns were reevaluated in light of the visits. It was at this point that a plan was agreed upon: whether it would be referral to a community agency for therapy for the child, family or marital counseling, a special school plan, continuation in therapy privately, or using new-found knowledge and advice to work on the problem by themselves.

Although a parent conference concluded the psychological consultation, continuing responsibility for the care of the patient rested with the pediatrician. Families were encouraged to meet with the pediatrician following their conference to discuss the suggestions offered. At times the pediatrician took part in the conference with the parents. Whenever a school plan was made, the pediatrician discussed the suggestions not only with the parents but also with the appropriate school personnel. Communication between myself and the pediatrician was almost instantaneous and verbal reports were amplified later by a written report. Although the bulk of the time was spend in direct patient contact, other services emerged during the program.

**Curbstone Consultation**

Parents frequently asked the pediatrician about child-rearing practices, child development, etc. In turn, they checked opinions with me. This consultation was readily available either by a brief discussion in the office or by a telephone call. For example, a two-year-old began evidencing regressive behavior (return to baby talk, temper tantrums, and negativism) as the result of a sibling in the house. When the mother was in the examining room, one of the pediatricians discussed the mother's concern with me and was then able to be supportive and reassuring to the mother regarding the reactive nature of the difficulties.

On occasion the pediatricians became involved in rather brief counseling with some of their patients (often adolescents). Opportunity for discussion around counseling cases that the pediatricians were seeing, especially when progress seemed to bog down, was made available. For example, counseling a very quiet thirteen year old who talked occasionally about fishing and other unimportant subjects was frustrating for one pediatrician. He was helped to look upon the boy's silence in a different light; he was being used in a different fashion than expected (as an accepting nonjudgmental adult with whom the boy could discuss something that he was interested in rather than conforming to adult interests). By accepting the boy's passive-aggressive manifestations of hostility, the pediatrician found that the basis for a different type of relationship could be established.

**Education Regarding Psychological Testing**

Periodic meetings of a didactic nature were held in which the pediatrician was able to learn about some of the instruments used by psychologists. We discussed relatively new psychological instruments as well as standard intelligence and projective tests. At these meetings the pediatrician reciprocated by familiarizing me with information about medication. My research skills were also available to the pediatric practice. The group became interested in designing more extensive screening of preschoolers. They were interested in the physical and also the social, intellectual, perceptual, and emotional areas. We spent many hours together thinking about appropriate tasks and evaluation techniques.

**Expanding the Network**

Although the major method I used for answering questions raised by the pediatricians involved psychological tests, the service was not conceptualized as psychological testing but as diagnostic and consultative service for the families served by the pediatric practice. A major element of the linking strategy is good communication among the groups to be linked. When working with children, it is important to include the school within the communication net. The pediatrician was in a position to communicate my findings to the school and since a good relationship existed between them, this increased the probability of the recommendations being carried out. As I became more acquainted with school personnel, I began handling more of the school feedback directly. Of course, this gave me a number of new referral sources who began referring directly to me.

Although the evaluations were carried out in the pediatric office, at times I would see families at other offices, especially if we were to continue in psychotherapy. When adolescents were involved, I encouraged the entire family to come, especially at the concluding feedback session.

Although the child-oriented psychologist can readily link up with pediatricians, others can pursue linking with similar success. A number of social worker colleagues have successfully linked with pediatricians. Their major focus has been running educationally oriented parent groups. This evolved into casework, marital, and family counseling. Another colleague, whose part-time practice consisted mainly of psychological assessments, linked up with counselors at the New York State Office of Vocational Rehabilitation.

Yet another colleague, whose major expertise is psychotherapy with adults, has worked out a linking relationship with a group of attorneys who specialize in divorce. The possibilities are limited only by one's initiative and creativity. The only major pitfall of linking is a complacency in the marketing area. Even when you link up with a large group practice and in effect have a number of different referral sources, it is wise to continue, perhaps to a lesser degree, to market yourself. Continue with community talks, continue to let the media know about your professional contributions.

Once you have established a successful professional relationship with a referral source or have linked up with a group, then teaching-oriented reports are not necessary. You can begin to take advantage of the dividends accrued as a result of your early time investments. A rapid feedback form, such as is presented in Exhibit 5–5, can be comfortably substituted for the lengthy teaching-oriented reports or the narrative reports usually sent.

## SUMMARY

Linking and teaching-oriented feedback via conference or report are two major ways clinicians in independent practice can mesh clinical practice and marketing for new business. It is the meshing of good clinical practice and inoffensive yet assertive marketing that is the benchmark of the successful private practitioner. Feedback that embraces much of what has been discussed in this chapter will be the focus of the next chapter. We will look in detail at the multifacets of feeding back information to both referral source and client.

**Exhibit 5–5** Quick Feedback Form

*Client Identification and Referral Question*

*Attitude toward Evaluation*
1. Distressed—anxious, depressed
2. Overtly hostile to procedure
3. Inattentive and distractible
4. Cooperated in matter-of-fact manner
5. Worked in eager and enthusiastic fashion

*Intellectual Level*
1. Significantly below average (retarded)
2. Slightly below average (slow)
3. Average
4. Significantly above average

*Emotional Reactivity*
1. Anxious and fearful
2. Dependent
3. Hostile or resistant
4. Balanced

*Emotional Development*
1. Immature
2. Age appropriate

*Diagnostic Formulation*

*Recommendation*

Chapter 6

# Marketing through Feedback

# 6

Feeding back information is a highly complex process that calls upon the practitioner's skills as a clinician, teacher, and business person. In the preceding chapter, teaching-oriented feedback was suggested as a way of answering referral questions to make you stand out from "the rest of the pack."

Referral sources, however, are not the only people who receive feedback information from clinicians. The clients you serve, especially early in the relationship during the evaluation phase, require good feedback; and you as a practitioner require feedback from your referral sources and patients regarding the effectiveness of your clinical practice and intervention strategies.

In this chapter we will continue our discussion of feeding back information to referral sources and then consider two other major areas where good feedback can make the difference between success and failure: feeding information to your clients and obtaining feedback information from your clients and referral sources.

## FEEDBACK TO REFERRAL SOURCES

It is a good idea to get in the habit of making contact with the referral source prior to seeing the patient. A brief phone conversation is often sufficient to give you some background information and orient you to the referral questions. An evaluation that is focused is more efficient and effective. Some practitioners have specific referral forms available for referral sources. Lewin (1978) has designed a number of referral forms depending upon the type of problem. Exhibit 6–1 presents an example of one such referral form.

I have found that a brief phone call prior to seeing the patient is sufficient. Informal surveys of referral sources have confirmed my suspicions that they prefer phone contact to filling out a written referral form. On the other hand,

**Exhibit 6–1** Sample Referral Form

STANLEY KISSEL, Ph.D.
1425 Portland Avenue
Rochester, New York 14621
716-544-5220

REFERRAL FORM

Date ______________

Patient's Name ______________________ Sex ____________ Age ____________

Address ______________________________________ Phone ____________

*Please complete the following or attach appropriate records:*

Background Information: ______________________________________

______________________________________

______________________________________

______________________________________

______________________________________

______________________________________

______________________________________

Reason for Referral: ______________________________________

______________________________________

______________________________________

______________________________________

______________________________________

______________________________________

Is the patient under your continuing care for this problem? Yes ________ No ________

Is a written report desired? Yes ________ No ________

Referring Physician ______________________________ Phone ____________

Address ______________________________________

while referral sources are pleased with rapid phone feedback, they also want "something in writing for the record."

The follow-up form seen in Exhibit 6–2 is a helpful tool in letting the referring person know where the patient stands in reference to your service. This is especially helpful when the referring person is a physician and the referral is for ongoing psychotherapy. Remember that whatever information you send out carries your name and address and thus serves as a marketing tool.

---

**Exhibit 6–2** Sample Follow-Up Letter

Stanley Kissel, Ph.D.
1425 Portland Avenue
Rochester, New York 14621
Telephone: 716-544-5220

Re:

Dear
Thank you for referring to me. I have recently seen him/her and the parent (s) whom you referred on . My impressions are as follows:

In the event that you think it helpful to discuss these findings and recommendations, or to set aside a conference time for this purpose, please call me.

Sincerely yours,

Periodic feedback by telephone or mail is helpful, necessary, and appreciated by referral sources. A major complaint is that once their patients are seen beyond the evaluation, they do not receive any feedback regarding the progress of psychotherapy. It is a good idea to make a practice of sending a progress note every three or four months and a brief summary note upon termination.

When the referral questions center around diagnostic issues, then a complete report should be sent to the referral person. In the previous chapter a model of such a report was presented.

The main point to remember is to feed back information rapidly and usefully. The information will serve the clinical purpose and will keep your name as a reliable practitioner in the mind of the referring person. When you terminate with a client, remember to inform the referral source that the treatment has been terminated. The referring person is often involved with the patient over many issues and will continue to be responsible for providing care to the patient. The closing note can be rather brief and cover these areas:

- presenting problem(s)
- duration of treatment
- success of treatment
- reason for termination

## FEEDBACK TO CLIENTS

Most of our clients, be they parents of troubled or troubling children, a married couple teetering on the brink of divorce, or a stressed individual riddled with symptoms, consult us with trepidation and ambivalence. At some point in a series of evaluative sessions we generally take time to discuss our view of their condition and make some suggestions for change. The tools we use are as varied as the possible intervention plans we can suggest. The section that follows is based on an information-gathering schema that can be translated into meaningful charts or tables so your client can have visual as well as verbal feedback. Early in my career I discovered that groups I talked with were more responsive and had greater recall of what I said if I left them a visual handout, i.e., an outline of my comments, some suggestions for further reading, or a schematic diagram of some major points. This applies as well to individual clients.

Feedback conferences are often anxiety laden. Introduction of structure in the form of visual feedback helps reduce anxiety and focuses the client's attention on the points the practitioner wants to make. The following procedure incorporates teaching-oriented reports with some suggestions made by Joseph Richman (1967) on presenting diagnostic information to patients and their families. The techniques used to gather the information are psychological testing.

Much of the hesitancy to present test findings to clients has stemmed from concern on the part of many psychologists that the patient might be too fragile or uninformed and that the information would be harmful. Reviewing the literature on the subject, Richman (1967) concluded: "The client emerges as a rather weak being while the psychologist accepts the magical image of himself as someone in charge of great and dangerous secrets" (p. 62). I have found the clinical sharing of test information with clients beneficial and those clients who went into psychotherapy did so with greater understanding and motivation. When discussing intelligence tests with individuals I have found it helpful to use the diagram on the front of the Wechsler form. I give the patient his or her scale scores and indicate that in general most people score between 8 and 12. I also talk about the meaning of each subtest, highlighting strengths and weakness. In general I attempt to work toward creating a specific set in the client's mind depending on my objectives for the discussion.

When evaluation includes both intellectual and projective tests, I provide information about cognitive functioning first. Richman (1967) has presented a clear example of feeding back information in this manner. The following example is presented with his permission:

The following procedures are those which have proven most effective for the writer. The WAIS or WISC scores and the Rorschach psychogram are the basic data used in the counseling. After the test blanks have been placed on the desk or table where both the patient and psychologist can examine them together, a typical introduction would go as follows:

"I gave you many different tests, both of intelligence and personality, so there is a lot of material. Of course, these are only tests which are scored, and the interpretations are made from the scores. The interpretations could or could not be accurate. You are the best judge of that. I will show you your test scores and discuss the meanings. The chances are that they will speak for themselves.

The intelligence test is called the Wechsler Adult Intelligence Scale; it's really eleven different tests. Each test gets at some other aspect of your functioning, so the test as a whole is very helpful in seeing where you function well and in what areas you are weak. In other words, you get a kind of cognitive map of your mind."

The initial phase consists largely of educating the client quickly in a way of looking at himself and his cognitive and personality abilities and disabilities. I spend much time explaining how the intelligence test scores are derived and the function which each Wechsler subtest and Rorschach score presumably gets at.

After this didactic introduction I write out the actual test scores on a fresh scoring sheet, subtest by subtest, explaining the significance of the pattern that is gradually emerging, emphasizing the positive but by no means ignoring or minimizing the problematical. I avoid psychiatric or technical jargon. I do not report the total I.Q. score, and usually comment that with all the wealth of material in the pattern analysis the I.Q. score is unnecessary and even misleading. Typically, if the Wechsler shows uneven or inefficient functioning, attention difficulties, etc., I make the interpretation that something is interfering with the client's functioning, and maybe the personality tests can help find out what this is.

With the Rorschach, I show the patient the psychogram, and explain that scores on the left reflect one's inner world, those on the right reactions to outer stimuli and emotions, and those in the center represent reality. I point out indications of mature and immature strivings, the presence and extent of anxiety, depression, impulsivity, etc. When there is ego pathology in the form of paralogical thinking and impaired reality testing, I deal with this through an "ego-strain" score, which is simply the number of responses containing severely disturbed thinking and/or perception. I explain this score as indicating that when pressures and strains are great enough the patient cannot think straight or tell the difference between what is real and not real. (Patients for whom this interpretation is accurate react with relief and very often with a description of some of these experiences.)

After the account of the formal scores the patients are told that what they see is also important, although less so than the psychogram, and can be interpreted as an analyst would a dream. Looking at it this way, I continue, the following themes were the ones which stood out most in their record. I then summarize the major conflict areas, and their feelings about themselves and others.

There are wide individual variations, indeed, in my approach to the patients, which scores I emphasize, and which interpretations I stress. Each session is tailor-made to the particular patient or his family, and each one contains much academic information about testing and the nature of personality and intelligence. The method will be illustrated by a report on one case in some detail.

## Case Illustration

*Therapist Dr. Ida Davidoff*

Mrs. B. A., a 39 year old mother of four, was referred early in 1965 by her psychotherapist for vocational counseling, a recommendation which clearly caused her considerable ambivalence and fear. She made very tentative steps towards contacting me for an appointment, but postponed the meeting and did not call again until a year later, in 1966. After many minor obstacles she finally appeared for two testing sessions. She remained very anxious during the examination, and the experience was clearly a most trying one for her, but she did cooperate to the best of her ability.

She was administered a test battery consisting of the WAIS, Rorschach, Bender-Gestalt, and Figure Drawings. The WAIS and Rorschach scores are summarized in tables 1 and 2. A report was written for her therapist. The patient was then contacted and an appointment arranged to discuss the test findings with her.

For the purpose of illustrating the counseling process, parts of the report will be presented, followed by the transcript of the same material as discussed with the patient:

*Excerpt from test report:*

> "On the WAIS, Mrs. B. obtained an I.Q. of 108, derived from a Verbal I.Q. of 110 and a Performance I.Q. of 106. Aside from one very lowered score (Object Assembly), 6 of the 11 subtests were in the Average range and 4 were Superior. She did best on tests dealing with social comprehension and awareness, a result consistent with the Rorschach, which contained an emphasis upon social concerns. Her approach, qualitatively, might best be described as a decompensating obsessiveness."

*Excerpt from counseling transcript:*

> (The tests were introduced, as described in the section on procedures, and the meaning of raw and weighted scores was explained, using the Information test as a concrete example. The patient's Verbal WAIS scores were noted down, subtest by subtest, with a concomitant discussion of the meaning of each one and its relationship to other subtest scores. I summed up the pattern with): "So the picture is of somebody who shows superior learning ability and good reasoning ability, but falls down on things like number tests which have more to do with attention and concentration." (The Performance test scores were then noted, saving her superior Picture Arrangement score for last, with the comment): "That's a very big difference. When you get big differences, with some scores very much higher than others, you start thinking that you're not using

your abilities for some reason; there's some interference with them."

**Pt:** In the discrepancy between them?

**E:** When there's that much discrepancy.

**Pt:** And your analysis is that I—?

**E:** That there's something blocking and inhibiting you intellectually. You did seem very anxious about the tests. When it comes to being smart, apparently there's a great deal of anxiety.

**Pt:** Well, that goes back a long time. You see, I never studied too hard in school. When I did I could do well, you see, and all these years I've kind of wondered if I really had the ability to do this.

**E:** So you were very anxious and there was this unevenness in the test scores. Putting two and two together, maybe they're related. The tests also show an ability to get through college. The problem is not that of basic ability but the interference with attention and concentration, probably on the basis of anxiety....

**Pt:** Well, that's possible. I read a great deal, but I don't remember as much as, say, my husband does. I don't know why. I take generalities out of things rather than remembering certain things. Maybe this is just me, or maybe I'm just—(Laugh). (The patient is now questioning the reason for her difficulties, which created a good opportunity to go naturally into the Rorschach findings; and so we did.)

**E:** Fortunately, you took other tests also, and maybe they can help you understand the basis of these difficulties.

**Pt:** Good!

**E:** It's never just one test but the whole pattern of different tests that help us. Let's look at the Rorschach. (With the scoring sheet before us, Mrs. B. was given an explanation of the test determinants).

**E:** Would you like to see how you did?

**Pt:** (Laugh) That would be interesting.

(I began with R (41), which, I commented):

**E:** Shows a good amount of productivity. Even though you impressed me as a very blocked person there's something there once the block is eased up.

**Pt:** (Clearly relieved) Well, I must admit I was apprehensive about these things Is it not so that when you decide in your life that you, you know, what kind of person you are, what abilities you have, it takes—I think one is apprehensive? It's good to face things, but . . . I'd like to feel the assurance that I'm capable. I sort of feel that I am, but I'm not sure.

*Excerpt from test report:*

The Rorschach was highly ideational, even overideational, and revealed a struggle with the data which bespoke a harsh and dominant conscience. There was relatively little reaction to external emotional stimuli, and the pattern was dominantly withdrawn and introverted. As on the WAIS, the Rorschach also revealed decompensating defenses. The basic character struggle was that of an obsessive with borderline features. Although the pattern suggested a chronic borderline adjustment, the level of anxiety, tension and depression, and some indication of periods of sexual agitation, revealed some acute disruption at this time.

*Excerpt from counseling transcript:*

Her 9M responses were interpreted as "Brooding, thinking where you just can't stop; it's too much . . . (But it also) suggests a capacity for mature thought, and it goes along with an interest in people." (As for the FM also being high): "We're getting a picture, so far, of maturity and of immaturity, which suggests an inner conflict between the child in you and the adult in you, with a lot of both being there."

**E:** There's a picture here of emotional unpleasantness: a lot of anxiety, a lot of tension, and a lot of depression. Just what these stem from doesn't come through in the scores, but they're probably based upon long-standing frustrated needs from childhood that have not been resolved or worked out. As for the outer side . . . you can express your feelings in a controlled way and also do so impulsively, and that's a nice balance. If you're always controlled you're cold, and if you're always impulsive you're in hot water, but having both is fine. Except that the total amount is low compared to everything else. It is still an inner, introverted picture. That's what you predicted, didn't you?

**Pt:** Mm-hmmm.

**E:** So you had some insight . . . (I pointed out the high number of populars and repeat the interpretation of an interest in working with people. The patient disagrees).

**Pt:** The one thing I hadn't done is, uh, I'm so wrapped up with many things at home and many problems and so forth, that I really have not had much contact with, say, friends and people all my life, which I would like to have done, you see. I'm just starting now, but it has not been that way, and so it's difficult for me to know.

*Excerpt from test report:*

Her ego seems under more a strain than she can deal with, and as a result, there are eruptions of primitive defenses such as denial and projection and more archaic modes of thought and perception. Parts of the blot are combined in an incongruous, illogical way, with little attempt to apply a more reality-oriented judgment. Thus, one card is seen as a candle which has two pairs of human feet attached, dancing. Another card is seen as angry fish with legs and with flowers growing out of their heads . . . In all, 30 percent of her responses contained some indications of ego pathology in the form of archaic thinking, defenses, or reality perceptions.

*Excerpt from counseling transcript:*

**E:** The one other item showing a problem is something called an "ego strain" score, which means that under severe stress you can't think straight; you get disorganized. You can't interpret properly and tell what's real or not. That score was 12, which is also very high. So the test picture is of somebody who is under very great pressure, so much so that if you went to school right now you'd find it very hard to have your attention on objective demands. There are too many unresolved problems.

(I do not present the most serious pathology before placing it in the context of the total personality pattern. Similarly, with the dynamic content themes, I present the deepest layer of problems last).

*Excerpt from test report:*

The projective tests reveal a strong feeling of being different from others, unformed and/or malformed, and of not belonging . . . Many of her percepts express a feeling of being wrong, or not quite human. Her feelings of belonging to the human race also appear uncertain. Her self image has an elfin but not quite human quality. Card I is Little Red Riding Hood. Card II is little elves. Card III is a half human, half animal creature. Card IV has the dancing candle. Card V Satan. Card VII is an ugly god out of ancient history; and so forth. Such quasi-human percepts indicate a severe disturbance in her own sense of self . . . A prominent theme in her percepts is that of a large figure with several small figures attached. The last blot, for example, is seen as "seaweed . . . one glob with sort of pieces hanging off from it, floating around." Much guilt, depression and feelings of evil are associated with her resentment, her covert rejection of the maternal and wifely role, and her associated feelings of not being a fit woman. On Card V she saw, first, a dead butterfly with shrunken and crumpled wings, and then Satan with two birds perched on his shoulders.

*Excerpts from counseling transcript:*

**E:** (I repeated the analogy between dreams and Rorschach imagery, as described in the procedures section). Because these are just ink blots, you have to organize them in accordance with something that has meaning for you, some symbolic meaning. One of the themes that stands out is very interesting because it is just the opposite of what I said about your social interests. You express the feeling of not belonging, of not being accepted.

**Pt:** Can that be, the two extremes? Aren't they sort of contradictory?

**E:** Possibly. They are at least conflicting and distressing. The same contradiction shows up in the way you think about yourself, as somebody who feels distorted or damaged or not made right in some way. Yet on the other hand you also show a much more accepting self picture, where you see yourself as pixyish. I would say the contradiction stems from ambivalence about yourself, but it must show up in everything and everybody.

*Excerpt from test report:*

(This section contained what I considered the patient's central problem, the symbiotic tie to her mother.) She expressed a severely disturbed relationship to the mother figure, who is loved and hated, degraded and looked up to, but from whom she is never separated . . . It would appear that the primary goal of therapy would be an alteration in her own mother-child relationship.

*Excerpt from counseling transcript:*

**E:** The feeling of not belonging and of not feeling adequate shows up as an identity problem. In terms of being a woman, a wife and a mother you feel that you're not up to it. In your symbolism one of the themes is that of not being an adequate mother. Another similar theme is the feeling of needing a mother yourself, and of a very close attachment to her. The suggestion is that you have not made the separation yourself into an autonomous individual.

**Pt:** (Stutters and stumbles around for words). This means I would need a mother figure myself... And then you said about the separation, that there's no separation between the mother figure and myself?

**E:** You don't feel like an independent entity.

**Pt:** Well, you hit it on the head. All these things, they all add up. That's one of the reasons I've been seeing the doctor. And as you mentioned, I've never had the chance to really grow as a person. That's why she felt these tests would be very good. When I suggested them, my doctor thought they would be very good for me, to give me a little stimulus and interest and to know a little about myself. I mean they go along pretty much in many respects with what I'm understanding. I still have a long ways to go... and even though these things have been, because I'm going to her they have been a lot better. I can imagine what may have been if I had taken this test a year ago. I imagine these things can change to a degree for the person's personality. It would be interesting to know in a year or two how things could be.

*Follow up:*

The patient did have an argument with her mother the weekend succeeding the counseling session, but there were no other negative consequences of the presentation of the test results, if the argument were a negative consequence. In her therapy sessions she spoke positively of the test counseling, mainly about the reassurance it lent her that she was intellectually capable. The patient has since moved to another state, where she is enrolled for a B.A. in anthropology and at last report is doing very well.

**TABLE 1**

*Summary of WAIS Scores*

| *Test* | *Weighted Score* | *Test* | *Weighted Score* |
|---|---|---|---|
| Information | 13 | Picture Completion | 9 |
| Comprehension | 13 | Picture Arrangement | 14 |
| Arithmetic | 10 | Block Design | 9 |
| Similarities | 10 | Object Assembly | 7 |
| Vocabulary | 13 | Digit Symbol | 11 |
| Digit Span | 11 | | |

Verbal I.Q. 110 Performance I.Q. 106 Full Scale I.Q. 108

**TABLE 2**

*Summary of Rorschach Scores*

| *Determinant* | *N* | | |
|---|---|---|---|
| | | P=9 | |
| R | 41 | O=9 | |
| M | 10 | "Ego-Strain"=12: | |
| FM | 8 | F– | 4 |
| m | 6 | Fabulized | |
| F | 10 | Combinations | 6 |
| FC | 9 | Confabulatory | |
| FC | 2 | Tendencies | 2 |
| CF | 2 | Total | 12 |

*Note:* The Klopfer scoring system was used, except that all shading responses were scored FC and some percepts were scored for two main determinants when both appeared important.

Feeding back information in this manner helps strengthen some early bonds that are created during the testing or early intake sessions. The patient is helped to become more ego involved in the process and the clinician's wish to be of help is clearly communicated.

Such painstaking consideration to make the evaluative findings as clear as possible creates good will. These satisfied consumers let their doctors, lawyers, ministers, or school counselors—the people who sent them to me—know about my methods and their own satisfaction.

## FEEDBACK FROM REFERRAL SOURCES AND CLIENTS

When the majority of clinicians think about the effectiveness of their work, their thoughts quickly turn to outcome of evaluation. In other words, how effective is psychotherapy? There is considerable research literature concerned with the question of effectiveness of mental health intervention in both children (Cass & Thomas, 1979; Halpern, 1968; Levitt, 1971; Mellsop, 1972; and Robins, 1972) and adults (Bergin, 1975; Eysenck, 1965; and Wells et al., 1972). The results are inconclusive and confusing as the literature is fraught with claims and counterclaims. In the children's field what seems to be emerging is that therapy accelerates change and that the more efficient the treatment, the more accelerated the change (Bergin & Suinn, 1975). This conclusion is equally applicable to work with couples, families, and individuals.

Although practitioners are accused of dragging their feet when it comes to bringing their clinical service in line with "the latest research findings," such findings are often ambiguous, contradictory, and not helpful. It is also important to remember that the research studies are based on probability statistics of groups and are thus not very helpful in the decision-making process of the clinician as he or she is faced with the daily responsibility of making treatment plans; nor is the research literature helpful when it comes to answering clients' questions regarding the effectiveness of *your* treatment.

The independent practitioner, however, needs to be concerned with the satisfaction of clients serviced and his or her effectiveness. Accordingly, the independent practitioner does a service to the profession, the clients served, and the practice when the service provided is evaluated. Regardless of the effectiveness of any therapeutic intervention, if the recipient does not feel some benefit, then the value of the treatment can be questioned.

I have made it a practice to routinely survey a sample of clients every few years. The survey form has been kept brief and a self-addressed and stamped envelope is included to maximize returns. The survey is conducted on patients I have seen privately as well as those seen at a clinic. The form is entitled "Confidential Questionnaire to Evaluate Clinical Services." I introduce the questionnaire by stating that I am interested in determining ways of improving my services. The questionnaire consists of five questions regarding the effectiveness of the services rendered:

1. Do you feel I was of help to you? Yes ____ No ____
2. (When a child is seen) Do you feel I was of help to your child? Yes ____ No ____
3. If you answered yes to question 1 or 2, in what way or ways was I helpful?
4. In what way or ways do you feel I can improve my services?
5. Would you or have you recommended my services to a friend? Yes ____ No ____

Using this type of format I have been able to gain feedback on the value of short- and long-term child therapy (Kissel, 1974), group psychotherapy, and day treatment intervention for children. In one survey, a clinic population of 168 children, I discovered that parents felt there was no difference in the effectiveness of the service they received whether their children were seen in long-term or brief psychotherapy. Staff at the clinic believed outcome was better when clients were involved in long-term therapy.

A major criticism leveled by parents in an early survey was that they didn't get enough advice and specific answers to their questions. This criticism was conspicuously absent in the survey done a few years later. Parents also want symptom relief for their children and improvement in parenting skills for themselves. This feedback information helped me to become more direct in counseling, quicker to give advice when appropriate, and to introduce new services such as educationally oriented parent groups. It also pointed out a need for me to become more familiar with intervention modalities that I was not trained in when attending graduate school, i.e., behavior and cognitive management. In addition, I found out that I had effectively helped 80 percent of the clients surveyed, which was personally very satisfying and also helpful when answering clients' questions regarding effectiveness.

In a less formal way I have surveyed my referral sources to see whether they were pleased with the feedback they were receiving (reports, phone contacts). It is also helpful to annually review your referral sources. The more information you have regarding which referral source is sending you clients, or who has stopped sending you clients, the better position you will be in to design marketing strategies aimed at a particular referral source. Remember, the most successful businesses are those that devote ample resources to "research and development." For the independent practitioner, this translates into investing some of your precious time in gathering feedback information from clients and referral sources.

## SUMMARY

In this chapter we discussed ways of feeding back information with both referral sources and patients. The emphasis was on the dual aspects of independent practice:

- excellence in clinical practice
- marketing yourself

Feedback regarding your own work is equally important. The chapter concluded with a discussion of getting feedback from clients and referral sources.

Chapter 7

# Marketing through Community Service

# 7

One afternoon a Roman emperor was entertaining himself at the Colisseum by feeding Christians to the lions. Several Christians were sacrificed and the crowd screamed for more.

The next martyr said something to the lion and the beast slunk away. Then a second lion: same result. And a third. The amazed throng began to shift its sympathies to the Christian. The Emperor announced that the Christian's life would be spared. He insisted, however, that the martyr appear before him.

"I am sparing your life," said the Emperor, "but before I release you, I demand to know what it was that you said to those beasts."

"I merely said to each lion: 'After dinner, of course, you'll be expected to say a few words.' "

As a mental health professional there is a very good likelihood that you will be asked to talk to some community group at least once during the coming year. The private practitioner should welcome the opportunity. You can contribute to the community you live in, help to dispel many misconceptions and misinformation the public may have on the topic of your talk, and, most important, *market your services and yourself.*

Most successful practitioners agree that talking to PTA groups, church or temple groups, local medical, dental, and bar associations, school faculty teas, and the like is an excellent way of establishing yourself if new to a community or new to independent practice. While established independent practitioners tend to be a bit more selective and limit their speaking engagements, they, too, see talking to community groups as good works combined with good marketing.

A good talk, like a good report, requires skill and planning. In this chapter we will consider how to become a community speaker and what goes into a successful talk. We will provide a number of successful sample talks.

## MAKING CONTACTS

Most community groups are "dying to get their hands on you." All you have to do is let them know you are available. The executive secretary or paid professional of local professional organizations can usually be found in the phone book. PTAs can be contacted directly through the schools; churches and temples are listed in the yellow pages.

A brief letter, such as the one presented in Exhibit 4–4, describing yourself and a selection of topics you are qualified to speak on will bring in some requests for you to talk; word of mouth will do the rest. It is strongly advised that when getting established and "soliciting business" you conceptualize the talk as a marketing strategy and make it clear that you are not charging a fee for this service.

Exhibit 7–1 is an example of a letter informing community groups of an interest in speaking at their functions.

**Exhibit 7–1** Sample Letter for Speaking Functions

Stanley Kissel, Ph.D.
1425 Portland Avenue
Rochester, New York 14621

Dear

I am writing to inform you that I am now available to speak with parents and educators on a number of topics relating to children and youth, their development, and their problems.

I have been affiliated with the Children and Youth Division of the Rochester Medical Center and am also in private practice.

I would be most interested in talking on the following topics:

..... Hyperactivity and Learning Disabilities
..... The Effects of Divorce on Children
..... Childhood Depression
..... Communicating with Adolescents

I look forward to working with your group.

Sincerely yours,

Stanley Kissel, Ph.D.
Diplomate American Board of
Professional Psychologists, Inc.

## NUTS AND BOLTS OF SPEAKING ENGAGEMENTS

Robert Haakenson (1962), of the Public Relations Department of Smith, Kline and French, has a number of well-chosen ideas on how to go about giving a successful talk. What follows is based upon these views. He suggests that the most important element of a good talk is *"having something worthwhile to say."* Three things to keep in mind when preparing a talk are: "meat and potatoes, tell, tell, tell and conversationality."

### Meat and Potatoes

In a well-planned talk we develop a single theme, that is, we talk about a single subject. We develop our theme with "specifics": specific examples, illustrative anecdotes, definitions, comparisons, contrast, and statistics. These are called the "meat and potatoes" of speaking. When the last vote is counted, it is the amount and quality of "meat and potatoes" that will determine how well an audience liked the speaker.

For our "meat and potatoes" we must do research. First we must reflect, that is, summarize what we already know on the chosen topic. Second, we must read—as extensively as possible. Third, we must converse. We can discuss our subject with everyone who is willing to talk about it.

We should gather at least three or four times as much material as we can possibly include in the talk. Then we can select the best items on the basis of (1) relevance, (2) accuracy, and (3) human interest. We know that people like stories. "Once upon a time" is one of the most magic phrases in our language; "for instance" is another. People also like action or motion, conflict, novelty, and the familiar with a new twist. These are the elements of human interest. A special kind of "meat and potatoes" is audio-visual aids: photos, drawings, graphs, charts, models, objects, tape recordings, visual recordings. Blackboards and projectors are useful devices. When properly used, audio-visual aids enhance a talk because they clarify meaning, give it impact, heighten interest, and spark the speaker's delivery.

Use of a molecular model in a talk about the structure of the mind illustrates many of the principles of effective visual aids:

1. It is an aid: it does not make the talk an oral aid to a visual presentation. A good test here is, can the talk be given satisfactorily without the aid yet be better because of it? In this case, it could.
2. It is simple; a few red, black and yellow wooden balls connected by dowels to form a structure symbolizing the three levels of the mind.

3. The visual is in sight only when being referred to. Easily available when its turn comes, it is equally easy to put down out of sight, making the point with economy and impact.
4. The molecular model almost automatically achieves effective display. It is natural for the speaker to want the audience to see how the model is assembled. Attention is focused on a unified image of visual integrated with speaker.
5. The visual incorporates action. Adding to or taking away from the aid heightens interest; marking up a map or graph achieves the same effect.

The following are some guidelines for effective visual-aid usage.

- Use a modest number. A good rule of thumb is one aid per main point. No talk should have more than five main points, and three are usually sufficient.
- Use a variety of visuals, i.e., a statistical chart, a map, a model, an actual object.
- Stow the visual out of sight when not in use. Otherwise it is a distraction, competing for attention. Handouts, a very useful visual aid, should be distributed after the presentation. Be sure your name and address are clearly printed on the top of the handout.

**"Tell, Tell, Tell"**

People sometimes argue over which is the more important: what a speaker says or how he or she says it. Often they fail to take into account that there is a third element that can improve both the what and the how: the way the talk is put together. Effective organization can make a mediocre speech good and a good one better.

How do we go about organizing the speech? Follow the rules for successful teaching: first tell them what you are going to tell them and tell them. Then tell them what you've told them.

The following simple outline can be adapted to almost any talk:

I. Introduction
  A. Icebreaker
  B. Preview
II. Body
  A. Theme or thesis
    1. Main point 1
    2. Main point 2
    3. Main point 3
III. Conclusion
  A. Summary
  B. Haymaker

What is an icebreaker? It is anything that loosens things up, opens the way for rapport between the speaker and the audience. Often the icebreaker is suggested by something happening at the meeting, a personal narrative, or a pertinent joke that will establish a common ground between the speaker, subject, and audience.

I have established instant rapport with parent groups by telling them about the conversation a pig and a chicken had one Sunday morning while standing in front of a restaurant. The chicken was feeling very pleased as she saw all the people come out of the restaurant looking very content and told the pig how happy it made her to be able to give so much pleasure to the people who had been enjoying their breakfast of bacon and eggs. The pig looked scornfully at the chicken and said, "It's easy for you to feel that way. You only make a contribution, but for me it's a total commitment." When the laughter subsides I remind the audience that professionals such as myself can only make a contribution while for them bringing up their children is a total commitment.

After the icebreaker comes the preview, telling in a few words what the speech is to be about. In addition to announcing the theme, it is a good idea to enumerate the main headings, the main points that will be developed. "I want to talk with you about the impact of stress. First I propose to outline the reactions of the body to stress. Second, I want to describe problems that can arise from chronic stress. Third and finally, I will suggest what can be done to combat stress."

Why have a preview since the audience will hear the speech itself anyway? Won't you destroy suspense? One purpose of the preview is to whet anticipation. It also helps understanding and retention, because it creates a frame of reference. Having a broad outline of what is to follow, the listener can fill in the pigeonholes, so to speak.

The preview should be as tantalizing as you can make it, but don't promise more than you can deliver. If you were to say, "Before I finish speaking I am going to convince every man and woman in this room that stress does not exist," I honestly doubt whether you could make good your promise.

In any case, the rule to avoid apology is solid gold. What a masterpiece of negative psychology to begin "Well, I'm really not prepared to speak on this subject . . ." If the speaker expects the talk to be poor, listeners will too.

How do we go about working out the main heading? The simple way is to employ time-honored speech designs. Here are a few:

- time sequence
  1. past
  2. present
  3. future

"The Gettysburg Address" is a famous speech organized in this pattern.

- topical order
  1. who
  2. what
  3. where
  4. when
  5. how
  6. why

  or

  1. political
  2. social
  3. economic

  or

  1. theory
  2. practice

  or

  1. animal
  2. vegetable
  3. mineral
- logical order
  1. problem
  2. damage
  3. solution

  or

  1. cause
  2. effect

In writing words to be read, we strive for smooth-flowing continuity but in speaking, conspicuous transitions are often desirable—even to the point of being abrupt or unexpected. The abrupt transition serves two purposes. First it adds variety. We may use the analogy of the composer bringing in a second subject in a related but quite different key. Second, since the logical place for a transition is between the topics you promised to discuss, the transition serves as a checkpoint for your audience. When you say "Let us now move ahead to the second area of discussion," listeners can see that you are making progress, that you are following a well-charted course, and that you won't ramble aimlessly all night.

An especially strong transition is a partial summation: "We see then that there is a mounting problem of discharged mental patients needing to make a successful return to the community. Now, let us examine the consequences if this problem continues unresolved."

Speakers, especially beginners, do well to emphasize the structure of their talks. One need not fear sounding mechanical, as if doing it "by the numbers." The speech needs a strong outline for the same reason a clay statue needs a metal armature; without this skeleton, the structure is weak and liable to collapse. Don't hesitate to preview not only your theme but also the main heading. Boldly enumerate your headings as you come to them. "Tonight I want you to join me in support of rehabilitation programs for former mental patients. First I will confront you with the problem that results from a blessing: the mounting number of discharged mental patients who must make the difficult adjustment to normal living. Second, let us consider the tragic consequences of failing to provide adequate supportive programs in the community. Third and finally, I will describe successful existing programs that require your support."

In the body of the speech, the speaker establishes his or her theme (or thesis) by developing main headings and embellishing them with "meat and potatoes"—specifics.

In the conclusion, the speaker should first offer a strong and complete final summary of theme and headings. Then the speaker can conclude on a note of triumph with a rousing haymaker, a hard-hitting, dramatic, and memorable crystallization of his or her theme. The haymaker may be in the form of a statement, question, quotation, poem, resolution, challenge, etc.

How long should a talk be? The best answer seems to be that of the veteran pastor who was asked by his new assistant, "How long should I preach when I give my first sermon next Sunday?"

"That's up to you," came the reply, "but we feel we don't save any souls after 20 minutes."

Most subjects can be covered reasonably in that time. The point of diminishing returns in the human attention span probably occurs within 20 minutes. A short speech will often permit a question-and-answer period and many speakers feel they can "score the most points" at that time. There are, in fact, speakers who believe the chief function of the talk is to be a springboard, stirring up questions and statements for the question-and-answer period.

**Conversationality**

Did you ever analyze what you are doing in a very animated conversation, perhaps a friendly argument? First of all you are assembling material. You are searching your memory for every instance, statistic, concrete example, or emotional appeal that bears on the argument. Subconsciously, you are also selecting material, choosing those arguments that are most forceful and convincing. You are presenting your arguments with persuasive gestures and vocal inflections and you are too interested in the reaction of your adversary—watching to see if you are winning the desired response—to be self-conscious yourself.

In short, you're communicating sound arguments forcibly presented. These are the essence of a good talk.

What sort of voice have you? Even if it's not good enough to get you into the Metropolitan Opera, it can be very effective for speaking. The most frequent fault of speakers is monotony. Vary the pitch of your speaking voice. Let it rise and fall to suit words. Notice how skillfully this is done by fine speakers. An interesting experiment is to play a speech recording, moving far enough away so that you can't make out the words, and just listen to the sound. Avoid the extremes of shrill screech or cellar rumble, weary plod or machine-gun staccato, mousy whisper or deafening blast.

A common fault of speakers is speaking too quietly. Speakers tend to sound louder to themselves than they do to their audiences. Speak up; don't be bashful. There is far greater danger of being too quiet than too loud. Anyone with normal vocal powers should be able to make himself or herself heard by an audience of 40, even in the midst of background noise. You can ask your audience "Can you hear me all right?" This, by the way, can be a very effective icebreaker.

How you look is as important as how you sound. Try to appear natural and comfortable. Mannerisms that call attention to themselves distract from what you are saying. Bodily action or physical expressiveness include movements around the platform, stance/posture, gesture, facial expression, and eye contact. Bodily action should be plentiful, meaningful and spontaneous. It is possible to have reasonable movement around a 2 ft. square platform even when hemmed in by program chairmen, president, head table, etc. Posture should be comfortably erect. An uncomfortable "West Point brace" and a slovenly slouch are equally bad.

Use gestures—just as you do in a lively conversation. Not only arms and hands but head, feet, and the entire body can make movements that emphasize the points you are making. Physical expression attracts audience attention, communicates meaning, and stimulates the speaker to be a livelier communicator in all ways. Meaningless thrashing about is bad, of course, but as beginners, we are far more apt to underdo than overdo. To get the habit of gesturing, a few awkward movements may have to come first.

Keep facial expressions alert and friendly. When we are nervous about making a speech, our fear tends to show in our faces as hostility.

One of the most important factors in communicating is maintaining eye contact with the audience. Eye contact should be direct and continuous. The speaker's eyes should engage all listeners in a sort of irregular sweep back and forth over the audience. Even when reading a speech, the speaker should be making eye contact with the audience 90 percent of the time.

By carefully observing these simple rules, almost anyone can be an acceptable speaker and a little more practice may turn him or her from an acceptable speaker into an outstanding one.

## The Wrap-Up

A good speaker knows that the task is not completed as the final lines are delivered. It is only as the last question is answered that the "day's work" is done.

Plan to have a question-and-answer period at the end of your talk or at some point while you are presenting your prepared talk. If you previously talked to a group on the subject you can anticipate some questions and be prepared with answers that will enhance the main point or points of your talk.

Your answers should be direct and to the point. You should not hesitate to take a partisan stand on a controversial issue but then you should spell out the reasons for your support of such a stand through the use of specifics. These add substance and conviction to an answer by amplifying and supporting it.

- *Amplification*
  - Definitions
  - Descriptions
  - Comparison
  - Figures of speech
  - Anecdotes
  - Visual aids
- *Support*
  - Case histories
  - Statistics
  - Statements by experts
  - Firsthand observations

In some instances it is helpful to document the specifics cited by revealing their source. This is called for when the information presented is hard to believe or when the audience appears skeptical about the speaker's argument. Documentation should never be a halfway job. It should include the name of the speaker or writer quoted, the place where the information was given or published, and the date and page number, right down to the context in which the words were expressed. In other words, chapter and verse, the works.

The use of supporting evidence probably is the most critical factor in determining a speaker's success in the question and answer. Do you have the facts? Or are you merely phrasing opinions in fancy language?

In every speaker's life there comes that awful moment when, to put it bluntly, you're stumped. When in doubt as to the correct answer, when you simply don't know, don't panic. Say aloud what you are saying silently to yourself: "I don't know." These can be the three most eloquent words in our language. The speaker who uses them need not fear losing the respect of the audience. If anything, they will admire you for your candor.

When you don't know and admit it, a good idea is to offer your own view on the subject, pointing out that your answer is inferred from related but not direct information. Another solution is to say "I don't know but I will be happy to find out and send you the answer." Or you may say "I'm going to ask one of my colleagues and let you know, if you'll give me your address. I'd like to know the answer also."

If you keep in mind the four major reasons for a question-and-answer period following your talk, you will be in a better position to field the questions that come your way.

1. It reinforces the main speech.
2. It increases the audience's knowledge.
3. It adds to the speaker's stature.
4. It provides valuable feedback information.

## SAMPLE TALKS

The remainder of this chapter will consist of three talks I have given, incorporating the points that have been suggested.

## Stress, Not Distress

I'd like to begin my talk today by telling you a story about Olaf, the caveman.

Once upon a time a long long time ago there lived a caveman by the name of Olaf. He lived in a dark dingy cave with his wife and two children. Every day Olaf would go out looking for food. Sometimes he would be successful and then stay in his cave until the food was devoured. One day Olaf was hunting for food and there descended upon him a giant dinosaur. Olaf's body began to prepare him for emergency action, the well-known stone or flight response. When the cortex of Olaf's brain perceived the danger, it sent a message down to the sympathetic branch of his autonomic nervous system, the adrenal glands. Under the influence of the body chemicals, Olaf's respiration deepened, his heart beat more rapidly, his arterial pressure rose, blood was shifted away from the stomach and intestines to his heart, central nervous system, and muscles; processes in the alimentary canal were inhibited; and the blood glucose level increased. All of these physiological changes, particularly the increased respiration, the redistributed blood flowing at higher pressure, and the increased number of red corpuscles set free by the spleen, which provides for essential oxygen and for riddance of acid wastes, serve to render the body more effective in the violent display of energy that response to danger may demand.

As Olaf's body was set with all these extra chemicals flowing, he was able to swiftly avoid the clutches of the dinosaur. It was dark by the time Olaf got home and the long walk home from Dinosaur Alley to his cave permitted his body to readjust itself as the running and walking used much of the processes that were put in motion.

Today Olaf is extinct, the dinosaurs are extinct, but what remains is stress.

While Olaf had many outlets for the body's reactions that were set in motion by threatening experiences, today we in modern society have no complete outlet for our stress responses and thus eventually we experience undesirable manifestations of the strain of stress, such as hypertension, increased smoking or drinking, irritability, depression, anxiety, sleep problems, heart problems, angina, migraine, ulcers, colitis, constipation, diarrhea, allergies, backache, tension headaches, arthritis, accident proneness, diabetes, and, yes, today even cancer has been linked with stress. These behaviors or symptoms that I have listed result from a condition that is really not a true disease in itself but rather a runaway condition of normal body physiological functions—the body's normal reaction to stress.

Economically, stress has been estimated by some to cause our nation over one hundred billion dollars annually. Much of the loss comes from decreased productivity, increased absenteeism, and general apathy towards work. In the economic marketplace these worker-related stress behaviors are called burnout; in the day to day social world these are called the symptoms of chronic stress. Regardless of what the label, stress is a strain on our physical and mental selves.

Stress is not necessarily bad in and of itself. We need a certain amount of stress to energize those mental and physical systems sufficiently to keep us alive and alert. Stress becomes a problem when it exceeds our normal level of available adaptive energy over a prolonged period of time. In other words, according to Selye, the noted stress researcher, stress becomes a danger and possible detriment to our physical and emotional health when it becomes distress. That is, when our bodies experience the physiological reactions of stressful events for a long period of time without appropriate adaptive behaviors. We respond to this state physically—by breaking down at our most vulnerable areas, whether the stomach, head, back, or other vulnerable spot, and behaviorally with response acquired from our parents and other significant adults in our background such as grandparents, teachers, ministers, etc. Such responses for example are anger, withdrawal, anxiety, depression. Ultimately our final response to the stressful situation is a combination: past experience, current physical reaction, and our self talk.

John Adams, another noted stress management expert, has suggested five major things you can do to combat the effects of stress and minimize it from becoming a state of distress:

1. Good nutritional habits. He suggests that one should have a sufficient balanced diet that contains an appropriate amount of vitamins, minerals, protein, complex carbohydrates, and fibers while minimizing consumption of sugar, salt, saturated fats, and chemical additives. In addition, it is helpful to have regular meals, maintain the recommended weight for your height and age, and make only moderate use of alcohol and caffeine.
2. Good exercise habits. Regular aerobic exercises help improve cardiovascular fitness while regular recreation exercise helps reduce tension and provides an opportunity for diversion and the development of outside interests.
3. Self-awareness. Begin to tune in to your own personal needs, preferences, and idiosyncracies as a way of minimizing situational stresses. The more you are aware of your needs, the less likely environmental situations will be overly frustrating. Practice assertive behavior and be prepared to stand up for your rights when you feel they are violated.
4. Letting-go techniques. In addition to good exercise it is important to become familiar with relaxation techniques and develop a good strategy for relaxation, whether it be meditation, muscle relaxation, prayer, visualization, or breathing exercises. It is also important to attempt to gain closure on work tasks and interpersonal situations, that is, finishing unfinished business and not letting it linger so it develops festering anxiety.
5. Finally, personal planning. Manage your time effectively from day to day and give some thought periodically to long-term goals be they social or career oriented.

Some other things you can do to help minimize the effects of stress are:

1. Improve your personal support system. Remember, no person is an island. In stressful situations we all can use friends and colleagues, especially those with whom we can be open enough to share ideas, fears, success, and problems. Like any important possession, support systems require care, attention, and maintenance, often difficult when under stress. Remember the old advice given to generals at West Point. No battle has ever been won by a general who neglected his supply lines and reserve troops. Don't forget yours.
2. Be increasingly aware of your self talk in stressful situations, that is, the tape recorder in your head that habitually responds to stresses. Separate the positive self talk from the negative and work on replacing the negative tapes with positive ones. The way you respond to any situation is in good part a function of what you tell yourself about it and how you feel about yourself.

In the 60s one of the major catchwords was "better living through chemistry." Although the emphasis was on the adaptive use of chemicals, many of our youth and young adults began to use chemical means to avoid the debilitating effects of stress, whether showing itself in the form of anxiety, depression, or especially boredom. While many of our citizens still use chemicals in combating the emotional effects of chronic stress, such as anxiety and depression, there has been a considerable increase in the use of nonchemical combatants of stress. Creative imagery, muscle relaxation, biofeedback, and diet are some of the more popular ways of controlling reaction to stress without chemicals. These help minimize the development of vicious cycles whereby stress energizes and then incapacitates the individual.

At the conclusion of our meeting as you are leaving, please pick up the stress inventory and carefully answer the questions. Should your answers to the questionnaire be excessively high, you might want to speak with your family physician or get in touch with someone at your local mental health center to consider how you can implement a personal plan to combat the effects of stress before they begin affecting you.

## Divorce: Its Effect on Children

Whenever I talk with a group I like to begin with a story, anecdote, or joke. However, our topic for today, the effects divorce has on children, is no joking matter. It is serious business. Currently, approximately 85 percent of all families are single-parent families and approximately two million children between the ages of three to thirteen, care for themselves. For the most part single-parent families result from divorce—not death or the new alternative life style. While it is customary to focus on the child, tonight I would like to consider the effects divorce has on the family, both children and adults; how it can interfere with a child's school functioning; and then conclude with some thoughts on what you teachers can do to be helpful to the child in the classroom. I also plan to leave some time for questions and answers after my prepared remarks, so please hold your questions.

A major error made by teachers and lay people alike when thinking about the effects of divorce is to construe divorce as an event. They make what I call the event error. For children the key time is the point at which the parents separate, whereas for the parents the divorce is a process. Rather than consider it as a singular event, one must consider the total process. First let's consider the divorce process for the adults.

The process for adults can take anywhere from two to five years and has been conceptualized as consisting of four major stages: deliberation, litigation, transition, and redirection. Let's consider each of these four stages as if they are separate and nonlinked.

### Deliberation

This is the time when the family is under much turmoil and one or the other spouse often decides he or she has had enough. While there have been usually many threats, trial separations, and what have you, one day one or the other spouse decides that he or she can't take any more beatings, or drunken escapades, or being responded to as if he or she doesn't exist.

### Litigation

This is the second stage and begins when one or the other adult decides to call an attorney and ends when the divorce papers are finally served.

### Adjustment

Adjustment is the time from the serving of the divorce papers until the adults finally realize they are no longer married and each is living as a single person. It is a transitional period fraught with much uncertainty, stress, anxiety, and depression. It is the time when the spouses, thinking a great deal about each other in their loneliness, often attempt to become reattached to someone else, live the life of a "swinger," and find it extremely difficult during this time to invest much energy or effort as a parent. It is during this period when the adult is most vulnerable to having poor relations with other men or women and often searches for a substitute parent for the child.

**Redirection**

The fourth stage is redirection. This is when the adults begin to feel at peace with themselves, see themselves as surviving in the present, and begin to have hope for a good life in the future.

Some dilemmas that face the adult when it comes to divorce are: what to tell the child, who should tell the child, and when to tell the child.

It is best to be honest and concrete with children, and, most important, reassure them regarding your continued love. Let them know that their routine will be minimally disrupted. During this period of time children often have questions about the affection of both parents toward them, i.e., if the adults stop loving each other, have they stopped loving the child? They are usually quite concerned and worried about who will care for them. They find their answers most often not in the words the adults give them, but in their actions—which need at this time to be regular and routine. The child needs constant reassurance that even though the parents have stopped loving each other, it doesn't mean that they have stopped loving the child.

When you as teachers come in contact with the divorced parent it's important to keep in mind that the parent who left fears the loss and rejection of the child's love just as much as the child fears the loss of that parent's love. As much as possible, it is important to have that parent involved in the child's schooling. Sometimes, a parent inadvertently gives the child a message that somehow the child can either reunite the parents or that it was the child's fault. A child may react to this feeling in school—he or she may attempt to be very good or very bad as a way of reuniting parents.

When teachers have conferences with parents who are divorced, the parents may attempt to place the teacher in the role of an expert or counselor, and often wonder what is best for the child in terms of their visiting. Keep in mind that the younger the child, the shorter but more frequent the visits should be. Remind the parents that notes, letters, and phone calls, but especially letters for preadolescent children who are in grades three to six, are extremely meaningful and important. The older child enjoys activities and going places. However, it is important to remind the visiting parent, often fathers, that they just don't naturally spend two to four hours a day entertaining their child, and thus that is an unnatural thing to do during a visit.

It is also important for the custodial parent to be aware that he or she is often the one who gets "dumped on" by the child. Such "dumping" leads the custodial parent, most often the mother, to see herself as a "poor wife and mother." She begins to blame herself for any problems the child may have. This just leads to a worsening of the parent-child relationship. Teachers can emphasize the positive side of the child and help the parent to think about finding external supports, such as community groups or extended family for the child.

Let's consider, specifically now, how divorce affects children. We have to think of three major factors when we attempt to understand the effects divorce has on children: the predivorce environment, the developmental stage of the child, and the reactions of the adults.

### Predivorce environment

Often, parents who divorce provide children an environment filled with strife, arguments, and abuse. When this is the case, more often than not children feel ambivalent about the divorce. On the one hand they feel positive that much of the turmoil is finished, yet on the other hand there is a longing for the parent who has left. The more overt harmony there was between the parents in the predivorce environment, the more overt sadness, confusion, depression, and unhappiness the child shows.

### Developmental Stage

Early school-age children (kindergarten through second grade) tend to show upset in the form of regression of body functions, mourning, and open expression of sadness. They do a lot of fighting and making up in play activity, as a way of simulating what took place in their environment.

Older school children, grades two to six, show more surface denial and yet feel a lot of shame—at times they believe that they have somehow caused or contributed to the divorce. There is a sense of differentness, that is, the child feels different from his or her peer group, even though realistically there may be children in the class in the same boat. When regression occurs in these children it usually attacks school achievement. Headaches, stomachaches, school refusal, and overt anger at parents are other symptoms of this period. These children tend to show more aggression toward their peers and seem preoccupied at school—often harboring worries that something may happen to the custodial parent.

Adolescents tend to show more pseudomature behavior and attempt to take on airs of being a substitute parent. They also sometimes act out in the community in terms of promiscuity, vandalism, and stealing. Many divided loyalties are experienced by youngsters at this developmental stage.

One of the most common questions adults have is whether it is better for the child for them to remain married or to seek a divorce. It is important for you to be aware that divorce is not automatically disruptive. It is traumatic, scary, disjointing, but the marriage that divorce brings to an end may have been more disruptive and disturbing for the child than the divorce.

Parents must make it clear to the child that they will not reunite; that the child is not to blame for the divorce; that disruptions of routine will be minimized; and if the parents are consistent in visitation (and do not use the child as a pawn to get revenge or express their anger and disappointment), then the child has a much better chance of adjusting to the divorce. Researchers have found that it takes approximately one year for children to begin to show they are coming out of the upsetting effects of a divorce.

In school, children feel less insecure when and if they know they are not different. Thus, discussions about divorce and separation can help children begin to realize that they are not alone.

Choice of books is another important area where some of the material that is presented in the context of traditional families can be presented in the context of single-parent families.

Sending invitations to attend conferences to both parents whenever possible is also appreciated by parents who are divorced. Finally, when children show some disruptive behavior, do not be hasty to introduce change in their programs or subject them to additional teachers. Try to keep their school environment constant for a while longer.

I have touched on what I believe are the key issues to keep in mind when attempting to be helpful. Some of you may have some specific questions or thoughts on areas that I have not mentioned. At this point I would like to open the meeting for general discussion.

## Discipline Is Good Sense

While thinking about how to begin my talk, I was reminded of the following story involving a chicken and a pig. On a sunny Sunday morning, the pig and chicken were strolling down the street and stopped in front of a restaurant where many people were coming out in a very happy mood. In the window of the restaurant was a big sign: "Breakfast Special—Juice, Coffee (and in big letters), Ham, and Eggs."

The chicken with a great big smile put her wing around the pig and told him how happy they both should feel for giving so much joy and happiness to people. The pig, with a sneer on his face, looked at the chicken and said, "It's easy for you to talk. You just make a contribution to this happiness. But for me it's a total commitment." Parents and professionals share a similar relationship when it comes to thinking about child rearing. I speak tonight with the clear realization that it is the parents who are totally committed to their child's upbringing and involved with day to day struggles, whereas the professionals make suggestions that do not have to be implemented.

One of the most complicated and difficult jobs facing people today is being a parent. Training in terms of formal education or apprenticeship is available for almost every type of work except for the job of parent.

It is a well-accepted fact that in order for children to thrive they need love and affection, just as a plant needs the warmth and light of the sun. However, as sunlight has to be supplemented by water for a plant to develop, so does a child need discipline from parents along with their tender love and care to enhance growth and development. Faulty discipline that is too much, too harsh, or not enough—coming from worried, not unloving parents who fear their child will be led astray, or develop poor morals, or get into trouble because of bad friends—generates rebellion and undermines good family relationships.

While most parents bring love and affection to the child-rearing process, they are often unknowledgeable as to the task of discipline. This task places a strong burden and responsibility on parents. Often they mistake the idea of biological capabilities, that is, the ability to bear children, for social wisdom, that is, the ability to bring up children. It is natural for parents to look to outside sources such as the media, books, and professional experts, pediatricians, clergymen, and child psychologists for advice and direction. Unfortunately, the advice often leads to confusion rather than to clarity. A poster I recently saw in a bookstore in Rochester vividly describes the dilemma of parents seeking advice. The poster read: 1910—Spank them. 1920—Deprive them. 1930—Ignore them. 1940—Reason with them. 1950—Love them. 1960—Spank them lovingly. 1970—(in big, bold letters) To hell with them.

It's clear that today's parents are angry about their inability to discipline their children. The anger often masks hurt and disappointment stemming from a lack of confidence in their ability to be successful parents. At times parents berate their child out of their own guilt—"I'm a terrible parent." In part, this has resulted from our high technological society, which often overemphasizes procedures and techniques rather than goals and aims. Tonight, I'd like to share some views regarding the process and purposes of discipline and some ways of achieving these aims.

I believe that discipline makes good sense. I purposely thought of good sense rather than common sense, and as I talk my reasons will become clear.

The first thing one has to have is a guiding philosophy. Often parents have different goals when attempting to discipline their child. At times the goals are hidden. Sometimes the parents feel they must change the child's action immediately and at such times pain or punishment is used. Punishment in the form of yelling or hitting is also used when the child "won't listen." The goal appears to be breaking the child's will, and often the child is compared to an animal. Discipline is used as a means to show the child who's boss. At other times the aim is to make the child into something different from his or her parent. Children are told they should be seen and not heard or they should do as they're told and not as their parents do. Issues such as smoking, drinking, and dieting are areas where the aim is to make the child into "something better—different—than the parent" and when punishment is often used.

One of the problems with using punishment as a technique has to do with the fact that parents usually use physical punishment because they wait until they've had it "up to their necks" and tend to punish impulsively and angrily—hitting their child. The child stops doing whatever he or she has been doing and unfortunately parents learn that this is the appropriate and only way to get their child to stop the behavior. The sequence unfortunately returns and more often than not it is the parents who are being disciplined by the child—that is, they're being trained by their child to act in ways that are not really helpful, and, furthermore, into becoming parents that they do not really want to become. In a sense, they become ogres, Frankenstein monsters, created and under the control of their little children. Punishment also has certain side effects, as do most techniques. The parents often get punishment in return; the child learns to yell and become aggressive, to model the behavior of the parents when frustrated. Finally, little long-lasting gains occur.

The true goals of discipline are teaching, guiding, and controlling those who are less mature, have less knowledge, and are easily upset and overwhelmed by their wishes, daydreams, impulses, and needs. To make life safe and secure so that children can grow up is the primary aim of discipline. It is not to shame the child, or to excessively punish a child, or to get even with a child. After instituting a disciplining method, ask yourself did I help my child in terms of teaching and guiding or did I attempt to shame, get revenge, or hurt him or her?

In order to discipline your child appropriately, you have to be organized, and have some preconceived ideas about how you'll handle discipline situations. Often when all goes well it doesn't matter what you do, or so it seems. What about these times?

- "Whenever the phone rings it seems that's a sign for my child to yell, want my attention, or for the kids to get in a fight."
- "Mornings in my house are a zoo, especially getting the kids ready for school. No one seems to know just what clothes to wear or what they're having for breakfast or who they want to go home with after school."
- "The house seems quiet until both children are in the same room and then the family ritual of brothers' fighting begins."

Often there are many recurrent situations that are ready made for strife. If you know how you will respond, it can eliminate much grief. It's important then that you have some plan of how you might handle the usual situations, which, of course, involves consistency but much more. Know what to expect from children. For example, young children require more attention and physical care but demand considerably less freedom and responsibility; older children want more freedom and less physical closeness. Budget some individual time for each child in the family. If you give them this, they won't have to demand it. For example, for the very young child find time to read a story, talk things over, just be together. As the child gets older, you can go out for a meal, just the two of you, take walks, for those athletically inclined, jog or bike together. Time budgeted for specific children will make it less likely that they will try and steal time from you.

When disciplining your child remain on target. Talk with your child in the present about something he or she has done in a clear fashion. Help the child to express a thought or feeling about something that's presently on his or her mind. Stay with the child's behavior. Criticize, correct, and reprimand about a rule that is being broken rather than about how she always spills or he never remembers to take out the garbage. Often we worry about and criticize the child for accidents, missed meals, minor cuts, etc. If we think about it, it's a miracle that our children survive beyond the age of ten. That they survive physical falls and diseases is testimonial to their strength and our caring.

It is the emotional climate that can do a child in. Negative emotional climate is like cloudy days. In a discipline situation it can often be avoided by staying on target.

Thomas Gordon, author of *Parent Effectiveness Training,* suggests parents often get carried away when communicating with their child and commit a number of sins. For example, they often order and command their child, saying such things as, "Don't you dare talk to me like that," or they warn and threaten their child by saying "If you do that then you'll be sorry." Some parents also commit the sin of being analyzers and interpreters of children's behavior, commenting that they're just jealous when they get upset with a sibling. Perhaps the sin most often committed is either lecturing, teaching, or giving logical reasons to children who are having difficulty or are upset; for example, telling children that smoking is dangerous or doing things for them that they're often quite capable of doing.

Instead of committing these sins, staying on target means a parent needs to listen to what the child is talking about with interest and show the child you understand his or her feelings. It is helpful to remember this when your child comes home either hurt or upset. In order to remain on target you can act like a mirror, reflecting the child's feelings. Remember, children learn about how their physical self is by seeing their reflection in a mirror and they learn about their emotional self by hearing feelings being reflected. For example, when a child comes home from school, storms into the house, and says how much he hates school because his teacher is a big boss and doesn't ever let him do anything, the positive response is "You sure seem upset," or "It sounds like you're pretty angry at school." The poor response would be "Come on, Frank, school can't be all that bad. If teachers are bossy it's because they have to be."

Staying on target also means avoiding labeling—when a child doesn't do something, it's helpful to discuss what he or she is not doing and is supposed to do rather than saying how stubborn, lazy, or dumb he or she is. By the same token, labels that are positive, such as "perfect," "sweet," "all boy," can also be harmful. Labels can blind you to what may be happening with the child and may lead to self-fulfilling prophesies. Children believe their parents and if they hear the labels often enough, they get absorbed into the child's system. Just as food is digested and absorbed into our bodies, so these labels get absorbed and then children begin to see themselves that way. For example, "John, have you finished your homework yet? You know you're not the brightest child." "Billy, finish all your vegetables. You're skinny enough."

Staying on target helps you to encourage your own feelings, sensitizes you to avoid labeling and criticizing your child, and focuses you on your child's behavior. When your child spills milk at the table, talk with him or her about the milk. For example, "When milk spills, we wipe it up," or "What happens when something gets spilled?" Not, "You clumsy—you're always spilling." If you want a child to do something, let him or her know specifically—she has to complete her homework before watching TV means she has to do problems 5–15 on page 10 in her math book and then she can watch TV. I want him to be happy equals I want him to be more affectionate.

Dependability is another important component of the discipline process. When the parents are dependable, their child learns what to expect and is helped to feel secure. This is what you've heard emphasized and stressed in the newspaper when you've read how important it is to be consistent in your actions, promises, and attitudes. When a parent is dependable/consistent, the child learns to trust; that is, to predict his or her parents' behavior with certainty. A child thinks "When I crawl into Mom and Dad's bed at night they will always return me to my room." A child thinks "If I throw food at the table, I will always be sent from the table." A child thinks "When I spill something, I will always be asked to wipe it up." This ability to predict with certainty leads a child to rely on his or her parents and the environment in which he or she lives. Children feel safe when they know what to expect. When children feel safe, they can explore their world.

Often, children test the ability of parents to be consistent in how they enforce rules that they make. The following scenario is quite common: (1) Parent states the rule. (2) Child tests the rule. (3) Parent gets angry, yells or hits, or sometimes overlooks broken rule in disgust. (4) Child feels insecure, that is, not safe. This sequence creates vicious cycles in parent-child relationships. The pitfall can be avoided by (1) Establish one rule at a time—it's forced exercise at becoming consistent. For example, let's look at establishing a bedtime rule: (a) Specify the time and be sure it's clear. With very young children you can tell them "When the big hand is on the 12 and the little hand is on the 8," or after a specific event, such as when a television program ends or after reading a story. (b) Enforce the rule every time. (c) View the child's protest in words or deeds as static or attempts to distract or test you. (d) When (c) occurs, ask your child what the rule is and if the child is unable to state the rule, then you repeat the rule.

So far we've been considering some of what you parents can do, but it's also important to consider that you have to feel satisfactions in order for discipline to work. Parents need to gain satisfaction from the relationship they have from their child. In order for children to feel comfortable with what their parents say, they have to believe that their parents are comfortable with each other and with themselves. In other words, relatively harmonious marriages and good adult-adult relationships foster positive discipline. A positive marital relationship encourages good parent-child relationships. When parents are upset with one another, they sometimes take it out on their child. When parents are unhappy in marriage they sometimes look to their child for satisfactions that they are not getting from their spouse. Tensions between the parent and child can lead to problems between husband and wife, which then exacerbates problems with the children. For example, a husband and wife agree that it's good for their child to go to bed at a certain time, but when the wife is alone she gets lonely and lets the child stay up later. The husband, when he is alone, gets preoccupied and forgets about the child's bedtime.

"Wait until Daddy comes home," says a frustrated wife to her five-year-old. Daddy cringes when the child runs from him at the door. Some parents require their teen-age child to give a kiss-by-kiss description of their dates. When a parent lives vicariously through a teen-aged child or a frustrated athletically oriented parent pushes a child to athletic heights, the child will feel exploited and becomes a prime candidate for a discipline problem.

Self satisfaction and marriage satisfaction are important cogs in the discipline wheel. They help to provide nonexploitative parent-child relationships. A child in a family where satisfactions are at a minimum might have the following attitude regarding doing chores: "They want me to be a slave and do things because they're too lazy." Another child might have a different attitude if the feeling of being exploited is not present: "Chores, dishes, lawn, etc., are not much fun but everybody does something and I'm glad Mom and Dad feel like I do them well."

In order to work, discipline has to be effective. Whatever you suggest be done or whatever you refuse to have your child do, you'd better be able to enforce. While it is the child's job to carry out a rule or do specific family chores, it is the parent's job to make sure that it is carried out. During the summer a child came in for supper before he completed mowing the lawn. Father said that the child must complete the task before supper and the child wanted to eat first. He sat down and refused to go back and finish the job. Father removed the plate, silver, and glass. The rest of the family—mother and sister—ignored the boy while he sat and alternately yelled and sulked. He then got up and returned fifteen minutes later, saying that the lawn was finished.

A boy's job was to wash the dishes before bed. The boy went to bed without washing the dishes. Mother went into his room, put on the light, and repeated the rule.

Remember: for effective discipline, especially when making rules, state the task to be performed, specify a time period, ignore irrelevant actions, and see that the rule is carried out. Rule violations that cannot be undone, such as coming in late, smoking, require asking the child to repeat the rule and that's it. It's simple and you have doubts, but it works.

The older your children become, the more freedom they have and thus they have to become their own "enforcers." The more reasonable and effective rules are at younger ages, the more children can incorporate them as part of themselves. Incidentally, a burst of rule testing usually occurs at transitional periods: (a) At around two and three when the child has good physical ability, can communicate, and is beginning to "become a person"—Dr. Spock's "terrible twos"; (b) upon entering school, where new friends are made, new tricks are learned, and new role models are found; (c) at puberty and early adolescence, when peer pressures and biological forces team up to push for independence and your child wants to forget how much the family is needed and the family does not want to be reminded of the child's growing distance from them.

Discipline has to take place *now*. A parent needs to stay in the present when providing discipline to a child. Children often try to avoid doing what is required by promising "later." Parents by the same token often worry about the future. Present-oriented discipline is like a savings account. It will ensure that there will be something for the future. Parents, on the other hand, not only worry about the future but also get caught up in the past. You have two time frames to avoid while the child has only one.

Let me give a few examples to show what I mean. A parent says "You have to be in early" and when the child doesn't obey, the parent thinks, "If I'm being defied now, what will it be like during the teen-age years?" Instead of considering whether (a) the time was inappropriate for the child, (b) what the worry was when the child was late, (c) what the child could do when late, (d) effective ways of enforcing the rule. Some parents view a child's not obeying as a personal attack and think their child is ungrateful for past sacrifices. Rewards should follow the child's action and not precede them: first you do your homework, then you watch TV; first you finish your supper, then you get dessert. Many times the child tries to put the cart in front of the horse and the parents are willing to oblige. "Just one more before" is a phrase I'm sure you've all heard. Discipline by staying with the discussion without reminding the child of past deeds or sacrifices. Avoid telling yourself, if it's bad now it will get worse later. Make sure the task is performed first and then provide the reward later.

Providing children substitutes when they'll be deprived of something they like, whenever possible, can help minimize frustration and teaches that when you can't get what you want, you may get second best, which is better than nothing. A common problem with two- and three-year-olds, especially when they're learning to crayon, is scribbling on the wall. Many two- and three-year-olds believe they're Picassos and want to paint murals. It's helpful to provide them with paper and pencil, letting them draw and telling them that walls are not for crayoning, scribbling, or writing on. Paper is. Then have them help you clean up the wall and after they've made their pictures on paper, display them. Repeat the procedure as needed in a matter-of-fact fashion.

Battles between brothers and sisters over rights are common when they're about two to four years apart, especially during the early and middle school years. Remind them that people are not for hitting and suggest that they can make a picture of the sibling that they're angry with and yell and scream at or jump on the picture. They can hit the picture—and it's important to provide this alternative form of anger expression—but not the person.

Swearing is another problem that occurs in middle-school-aged children. Swearing, of course, is a substitute—it's a substitute in words for action. But many times the words are worse than the action. Ask your child for a definition of the word to see if the word is used appropriately. Indicate that what he or she is really concerned about is anger. Provide a more acceptable word to say when feeling angry.

Using substitutes is often a way of avoiding prohibitions. When teaching a young child how to swim, rather than telling her to avoid deep water and possibly make her fearful of water, you can have her play in the shallow water with older brothers and sisters, or yourself, and therefore while she's playing in the shallow water, she cannot swim in the deep water.

Finally, it's important with any approach for discipline to be evaluated. Know whether you're achieving your goals. Are the kids growing up the way you want them to? Is the effort you're putting into a particular plan paying off? Are you giving your kids a chance to talk to you about what they think? Is there enough time for husband and wife to talk specifically about what pleases and displeases them with their family? A more specific way to evaluate your plans is by keeping a record of how often a certain action or attitude occurs, and seeing whether or not what you do to change it makes a difference. Do things get better, remain the same, or get worse?

I hope you agree with me that appropriate discipline, while hard work makes good sense; that is, (G) Know your goal; (O) Have an organized approach; (O) Remain on target, that is, remind the child about present behavior; (D) Be dependable—when you say something, consistently follow through; (S) Derive satisfaction from marriage and child relationships; (E) Effective discipline is realistic and enforceable; (N) *Now,* not the past or the future, is the major focus of the discipline process; (S) Substitute what is prohibited with something acceptable; and (E) Evaluate what you're doing. Keeping a record is one good way.

## SUMMARY

Presenting community talks is a successful marketing tool for establishing your practice. The nuts and bolts for constructing and presenting community talks were presented. Successful presentations on divorce, stress, and discipline were provided to illustrate the points made throughout the chapter.

Chapter 8

# Marketing through Education

# 8

Communication theory tells us that messages contain a covert and an overt component. The independent practitioner overtly educates the audience by giving information while covertly saying "I'm available as a healer should you find the need for one."

## BOOKS

Bibliotherapy, the use of literature to help people cope with the stress of loving, working, and child rearing via information and education has become a thriving therapeutic enterprise (Halpern and Kissel, 1976; Fassler, 1978). As we have suggested, clinicians giving talks in the community are wise to leave something concrete with each person attending. Annotated bibliographies of selected works on your topic, reproduced on letterhead stationery, will serve the dual communication purpose of education and marketing. The following is a sampling of well-received works and is not meant to be a comprehensive listing. However, it should be sufficient for most practitioners to choose a few titles in constructing a reading list.

### Practical Guidance for Parents

- *The Magic Years*. Selma Fraiberg. New York: Charles Scribner's Sons, 1959 (305 pages, paperback).

The subtitle of this delightful book is "Understanding and Handling the Problems of Early Childhood." The title does not indicate a sentimental description of children but rather that period when to the child so many things seem to happen without reason, "by magic." A professor of social casework, and for many years a practitioner in the field of psychotherapy with children, Mrs. Fraiberg presents scientific material in simple language readily understood by laymen, without resorting to "jargonese." She also has a special understanding of the inner feelings of the young child that shines through in her sometimes humorous but always sympathetic descriptions of experiences of early childhood. She discusses the many aspects of aggression and controls, fears and anxieties, discipline, acquisition of language, sex education, toilet training, and other subjects in practical terms applicable to daily living.

Although *The Magic Years* was first published over twenty years ago, the insights presented are still relevant.

• *How To Influence Children.* Charles Schaefer. New York: Van Nostrand Reinhold Co., 1978 (203 pages).

Dr. Schaefer draws upon a wide variety of approaches that have successfully been used to influence children. He presents 69 practical techniques to help parents manage and guide their children toward healthy growth and development.

The first section of the book covers such management techniques as rewarding, modeling, contracting, shaping, natural consequences, prompting, distancing, physical control, and limit setting. The second section, "Child Guidance," considers creative problem solving, reasoning, advice, value clarification, developing confidence in child rearing, clarifying children's roles, chores, failure, and constructive criticisms.

The final section focuses on ways to build positive family relationships: "How To Listen So Children Will Talk," "How To Talk So Children Will Listen," "Showing Empathy," "Loving Children," "Establishing Mutual Trust," "Individualize," and "Conducting Family Councils" are a few of the headings.

An appendix outlines some general principles of emotional, social, and moral development in children.

• *The Family Game: A Situational Approach to Effective Parenting.* Paul Hersey and Kenneth H. Blanchard. Reading, Mass.: Addison-Wesley Publishing Co., 1978 (227 pages).

The authors present a complete and systematic approach aimed at helping parents relate effectively to children in almost any situation—"from household chores and grades to swimming lessons and teen-age sex."

Knowing how to respond to your children in a variety of situations is the key to good parenting, say the authors, and they have developed a practical approach that will help you "grow winners." Using numerous examples and anecdotes, the authors explain how you can understand why kids behave as they do and influence them in a positive way.

First of all, you need to know the specifics of the situation you are trying to influence and then act in the most appropriate parenting style: "telling," "selling," "participating," or "delegating." For instance, Jackie may not require a lot of supervision when she's learning how to play tennis, but she might need a lot of attention and help with her social studies homework.

Hersey and Blanchard bring together in an easy-to-understand manner many of the currently popular child-rearing concepts and offer numerous strategies for using parenting styles to make effective day-to-day decisions about your children.

• *Problems of Parents.* Benjamin Spock, M.D. Boston: Houghton Mifflin Co., 1962 (308 pages).

This book is parent centered, concentrating on topics that involve the feelings of mothers and fathers—parents' quarrels, guilt about favoritism, resentment at interfering grandparents and difficult neighbors, and the inevitable frustrations of management problems. There are sections on facing facts with your child, including telling a child about death; talking with young adolescents about dating and love; coping with divorce, widowhood, and remarriage; and a final chapter giving Doctor Spock's answer to the question of whether we are rearing our children soundly in view of the world they face.

• *Between Parent and Child.* Haim G. Ginott. New York: Macmillan Publishing Co., 1965 (223 pages, also available in paperback).

Based on sound psychological principles, this book is written in a simple and specific style, offering concrete suggestions for meeting daily situations. It presents a helpful approach to conversing with children; new ways of praise and criticism, avoiding self-defeating patterns using threats, bribes, or sarcasm; responsibility and independence; permissiveness and limits; jealousy; sex education. There is also a chapter on some of the sources of anxiety in children and ways of coping with them.

In the final pages are descriptions of both children and parents in need of professional help, and references to sources from which such help can be secured. This book has been very frequently cited by parents as one they have found to be helpful.

• *Your Child Is a Person.* Stella Chess, M.D., Alexander Thomas, M.D., and Herbert Birch, M.D. New York: Parallax, 1965 (213 pages, paperback).

The interest of the authors in studying individual differences in children's behavior from infancy through the early school years, and analyzing temperament and its interaction with other factors, led to their N.Y. Longitudinal Study of Child Development, begun in 1956. From early infancy, such characteristics as activity level, regularity, approach or withdrawal as responses to a new situation, adaptability to change in routine, level of sensory threshold, positive or negative mood, intensity of response, distractibility, persistence and attention span were studied to describe temperament or preponderant pattern of functioning. The authors give practical suggestions for guiding healthy development, with examples of how children with similar temperament can evolve in one direction or another. Two especially useful chapters are "Establishing House Rules" and "The Difficult Child."

• *What To Do When "There's Nothing To Do."* Members of the Staff of Boston Children's Medical Center and Elizabeth M. Gregg. New York: Dell Publishing Co., 1970 (186 pages, paperback).

A book that may be suggested to young mothers who have had limited experience with small children, this resource contains hundreds of suggestions for play appropriate to the toddler and preschooler. Many ideas use simple materials available in every home. There are also lists of books and records that have proven to be especially enjoyed by young children.

• *What Teenagers Want to Know.* Wesley W. Hall. Chicago: Budlong Press, 1978 (126 pages).

This excellent book was written with the understanding that pre- and early adolescence can be a disturbing time. Dr. Hall introduces the teen-ager to what will follow by presenting a series of statements that cover most of the concerns teen-agers have. The first ten chapters focus on biologically related aspects of adolescents and cover such areas as becoming a woman, becoming a man, young mothers, preventing pregnancy, and venereal disease. Chapters on the interpersonal aspects of heterosexual relationships, feelings, drug use and abuse, and relating to parents are also included.

The great variety of material presented is useful; its presentation is made very real by the many examples and illustrations.

• *How To Survive Parenthood.* Eda J. LeShan. New York: Random House, Inc., 1965 (242 pages).

This thoughtful book written by a child psychologist who is also a mother could serve as an antidote or a reassurance to parents who have read too many books, have tried too hard to be perfect parents, or who have succumbed to the theory that everything that goes "wrong" in child raising is somehow the parents' "fault." There is more than a touch of humor in this book, but it also has a deep feeling about the need to gain new perspectives, to use new knowledge in such a way that "instead of paralyzing us it would free us to be more natural, more deeply and truly ourselves, to open ourselves to life, and to live by the heart as well" (p. 20).

There is discussion about the preschool years, the school-age child, adolescence and young adulthood, the concerns of working mothers, and the changing aspects of parenthood when the children are grown. In addition, this book has a particularly sensitive and helpful approach to some of the concerns parents have about adolescents and college-age young people in these times, with thought-provoking paragraphs about ways of keeping open the lines of communication.

• *Child Sense, A Pediatrician's Guide for Today's Families.* William E. Homan, M.D. New York: Basic Books, Inc., 1969 (308 pages).

Doctor Homan's book is different from many "guides for parents." It obviously comes from a tremendous amount of experience with children and parents and an equal amount of love and respect for them. There is humor in the book—a wit that prods the reader to pause and admit somewhat wryly at times: "*That* makes sense."

Doctor Homan points out that parenthood is approached by all parents with meager experiences and spotty knowledge; he says there is a striking similarity and repetition among the lessons learned by parents in family after family during their on-the-job training, with the same errors, the same finally acquired understanding. This provocative and refreshing book draws from his experience and that of his associates those elements that seem to repeat themselves most often and that seem to be most significant in helping or hindering the child.

• *The Adopted Family.* Florence Rondell and Ruth Michaels (Book I: *You and Your Child, A Guide for Adoptive Parents,* rev. ed. 58 pages; Book II: *The Family That Grew,* rev. ed., 20 pages). New York: Crown Publishers, Inc., 1965.

Book I has suggestions about preparation for adoption as well as a thoughtful discussion of questions the adopted child has from early childhood through adolescence. Book II, to be read to a young child, does not have the sugary sentimentality of some of the books intended to introduce the subject of adoption, nor does it overemphasize the "chosen baby" explanation. It includes a simple statement of life's beginnings and the "why" of adoption, which is missing from some of the other books on this subject.

• *Some Special Problems of Children—Aged Two to Five Years,* rev. ed. Nina Ridenour and Isabel Johnson. New York: Child Study Association of America, 1966 (64 pages).

This particularly helpful pamphlet was first developed as a joint project of two New York City groups, originally planned for use by public health nurses working with parents in well-child clinics. The intent was to give practical advice and a point of view about child rearing drawn from the wide range of thinking of authorities in many fields of child care. This edition has the following contents, with each section containing a discussion of the whys of the problem, the feelings of both parents and child, and finally some very specific suggestions on handling the problem with some dos and don'ts for the parent or teacher: when a child (1) hurts other children, (2) is destructive, (3) uses bad language, (4) won't share, (5) sucks his or her thumb, (6) still wets, (7) masturbates, and (8) has fears.

• *Between Parent and Teen-ager.* Haim G. Ginott. New York: Avon Books, 1971 (253 pages).

This book continues the developmental journey Dr. Ginott began in his previous book, *Between Parent and Child.* He suggests techniques aimed at making life happier for both the teen-ager and the parent, discussing many adolescent problems that parents face in their daily dealings with their teen-age children and then suggesting scores of practical and specific solutions.

Each of the 12 chapters, which cover such issues as anger, conflicts, rebellion, driving, drinking, drugs, and sex, is filled with models of parent-teen-age dialogue that are highly informative to parents as they struggle to communicate with and guide their teen-age children.

• *Liberated Parents, Liberated Children.* Adele Faber and Elaine Mazlish. New York: Avon Books, 1975 (237 pages).

The book was written by two parents regarding their five-year experiment in family living according to the principles espoused by child-centered permissive guidance experts. It is filled with observations, examples, actual dialogues, and practical living situations as these two parent-authors struggle with the stresses and realities of day-to-day living—and attempt to translate theory into practice. There are many very good illustrations of the type of communication Haim Ginott believed so important to building self-esteem in children. A most unique aspect of this book is the way the authors candidly discuss their failures, frustrations, and feelings in applying outsiders' suggestions on being a parent.

• *Children's Friendships.* Zick Rubin. Cambridge, Mass.: Harvard University Press, 1980 (165 pages).

Dr. Rubin combines the scholarly approach of a scientist with the warmth and sensitivity of a clinician as he provides new and important insights on how children go about making friends.

*Children's Friendships* covers such questions as how friendship develops out of the simple play among young toddlers, how the child's conception of friendship changes with increasing cognitive sophistication, how individuals become popular or unpopular and how this affects them, why children form cliques, adopt stereotypes, follow fads, and (almost universally) exclude members of the opposite sex in the years just before puberty. The author's answers to these and other questions will be very helpful to parents as they support and guide their children through their formative years.

- *The Politics of Adoption.* Mary Benet. New York: The Free Press, 1976 (364 pages).

This book demonstrates how numerous questions concerning adoption have been answered throughout history. The adoptive situation is examined from the point of view of the natural parents, the adoptive parents, the child, and the adoption agency. The book deals openly with the adopted child's need to feel connected to a biological past; the quest for identity, self-definition, and emotional maturity; and the conflict of when and how to tell children they are adopted.

**Sex Education**

*Books For Parents*

- *Dr. Spock Talks With Mothers—Growth and Guidance.* Benjamin Spock, M.D. New York: Crest Books (Fawcett), 1964 (272 pages).

Chapter 5, "Attachments and Anxieties Between Three and Six," is an excellent description in readily understood terms of the significant emotional developments taking place below the surface, and of the strains of unconscious rivalry in the Oedipal stage. It answers briefly and very specifically some of the most common questions parents have at this period of their children's growth.

- *What To Tell Your Children About Sex.* Child Study Association of America. New York: Pocket Books, 1968 (157 pages, paperback).

This book is written simply and directly, in question-and-answer form. The stages of child development from infancy through adolescence are each covered in a separate section. Especially useful is the information on children's questions and the questions parents ask about their youngsters' sexual growth. Other helpful features of this concise and well-written volume are a chapter called "Facts of Life Illustrated," with simple diagrams, a reading list for parents and children, and an index of childrens' and parents' questions.

• *Your Growing Child and Sex.* Helene S. Arnstein in consultation with the Child Study Association of America. Indianapolis: Bobbs-Merrill Co., 1967 (188 pages).

The subtitle of this book is "A Parent's Guide to the Sexual Development, Education, Attitudes and Behavior of the Child—from Infancy Through Adolescence." Included are chapters on how the baby learns about love, toilet training as a step forward in sexual development, learning to be a boy or a girl, how children learn to control their impulses, masculinity and femininity, and even a chapter about sexual behavior in the college years. Sections called "Summary Points That May Be Helpful" give excellent impetus to parent discussion.

• *Sex in the Adolescent Years: New Directions in Guiding and Teaching Youth.* Isadore Rubin and Lester A. Kirkendall, eds. New York: Association Press, 1968 (23 pages).

This fine book brings together the writings of 18 knowledgeable and skilled authorities on guidance in sex education for the adolescent. Some of the important aspects included are what real sex education means; what parents and teachers should know about teen-age development; what young people really want to know about sex; what teen-agers should know about anatomy and reproduction; helping young people establish standards and values; understanding the problems involved in premarital sex, unwed pregnancy, and parenthood; anxieties about homosexuality; and helping the development of the handicapped. Both of the editors are affiliated with the Sex Information and Education Council of the U.S. (SIECUS) and have had wide experience in family life education.

*Books for Children*

• For many children from 18 months on, a story time is a time of special closeness. There are scores of books to be found at the supermarket, drugstore, and 5-and-10 cent store, like the Wonder Books and Little Golden Books. A few titles in the Golden Books series will illustrate the kind of helpful and colorful (and inexpensive) picture books that may be found: No. 291, "The New Baby"; No. 340, "My Baby Sister"; No. 466, "Baby Dear"; No. 352, "We Help Mommy"; and No. 468, "We Help Daddy."

- *Love Is a Special Way of Feeling.* Joan Walsh Anglund. New York: Harcourt, Brace, 1960.

This little book is more philosophical. It depicts in a delightful way how small children can understand the very deep subject of human feelings of love.

- *How Babies Are Made.* Andrew C. Andry and Steven Schepp. Illustrated by Blake Hampton. New York: Time-Life Books, 1968 (88 pages, approximately half in color).

Designed for children ages three to ten, this book uses the unusual media of paper sculpture to show how flowers are fertilized, how animals mate, and finally how human beings conceive and bear their children. The scientific description of fertilization would not be understood by a three-year-old but the pictures would be, for the most part.

- *Growing Up, How We Become Alive, Are Born, and Grow,* 4th ed. Dr. Karl de Schweinitz. New York: Macmillan Publishing Co., 1965 (54 pages).

A well-known writer in the field of social work, Dr. de Schweinitz presents this material as a nature story, giving young children a picture of the total life processes we share with birds, fish, and animals. The book is beautifully illustrated with natural photographs and drawings.

- *Before You Were a Baby.* Paul Showers and Kay Sperry Showers. New York: Thomas Y. Crowell Co., 1968 (13 pages).

A Let's-Read-And-Find-Out Science Book, this is simple and clear with good illustrations by Ingrid Fetz.

- *Letters to Jane.* Gladys Denny Schultz. Philadelphia: J.B. Lippincott Co. 1965 (27 pages).

Recommended for middle and older teens, both this volume and the one mentioned above help young people find answers to their questions about sex and dating.

• *Boys and Sex.* Wardell B. Pomeroy. New York: Delacorte Press, 1968 (157 pages).

This book is written for adolescent boys, speaking frankly about the years of puberty and early manhood. It attempts to clear up the misinformation, myths, and fears that may disturb the healthy sexual development of the average boy.

**Divorce**

*Books for Adults*

• *The Courage to Divorce.* Susan Gettleman, and Janet Markowitz. New York: Simon & Schuster, 1974 (304 pages).

Written from professional and personal experience of the authors, this book presents a thought-provoking point of view about divorce today.

• *Explaining Divorce to Children.* Earl A. Grollman, ed. Boston: Beacon Press, 1969 (402 pages, paperback).

This is a compilation of articles about divorce, including different experts' social and religious points of view. A chapter called "The Father Question Hour" discusses the thoughts expressed by a very verbal two-year-old, described through his mother's diary about her responses and problems over a period of time. "Parents Without Partners" is another useful chapter.

• *Living in Step.* Ruth Roosevelt and Jeanette Lofas. New York: Stein & Day, 1976 (248 pages).

The realistic difficulties experienced by stepfather or stepmother are honestly presented. The book has many helpful practical suggestions.

• *Marital Separation.* Robert J. Weiss. New York: Basic Books, 1975 (334 pages).

Some studies have shown a protracted separation is potentially more difficult for children to cope with than a loss through divorce or death. This study of experiences and feelings of partners who separate is useful because it identifies common reactions and increases insights of those experiencing similar circumstances.

• *The Parents' Book About Divorce.* Richard Gardner. Garden City, N.Y.: Doubleday & Co., 1979 (368 pages).

This book provides an in-depth coverage of the major problems parents are confronted with when dealing with their children's reactions to separation and divorce. In the introduction to this book, Dr. Gardner states that he will not "provide any simple answers. The problems dealt with here are complex. Those who would give simple answers to these complicated problems may initially attract a wide audience; however, their solutions are doomed to failure and those who rely on them are bound to become disappointed and disillusioned." He goes on to discuss such issues as staying together for the sake of the children; maternal vs. paternal custody; how, when, and what children should be told; how to handle parental guilt feelings; and dating and remarriage for divorced parents.

Dr. Gardner's treatment of these issues is clear, well written, and sprinkled with sound practical advice.

• *Yours, Mine and Ours: Tips for Stepparents.* Washington, D.C.: Department of Health, Education, and Welfare, 1978 (27 pages).

This publication presents some observations made by stepparents about their experiences. It does not say all there is to say on the subject, nor does it include the advantages to be found in the stepfamily situation. It is designed to help new and future stepfamilies look more realistically at some of the problems that may confront them.

The conflicts and tensions that all families experience at times are complicated in a steprelationship. There are problems unique to the stepfamily. Many stepfamilies tend to be influenced, albeit unconsciously, by myths. The absent parent, living or dead, can be a source of tension. Emotional arguments arise relative to "his," "her," and "their" children; the family budget and ex-spouses; and differences in previous family life styles.

The concluding chapter, entitled "More Help and Information," discusses where to get help and offers some suggestions for further reading.

*Books for Both Children and Adults*

The following code is used to categorize the books described in this section:

B = Breaking Up Period
A = Aftermath of the Divorce
M = Managing Everyday Living

- (B,A,M) *The Boys and Girls Book about Divorce.* Richard A. Gardner. New York: Science House, 1970 (234 pages, also Bantam paperback).

Written by a child psychiatrist, this book discusses children's feelings about divorce, uses of love and of anger, the fear of being alone, getting along better with parents and stepparents. (Age 10 up).

- (B,A,M) *How to Get It Together When Your Parents are Coming Apart.* Arlene Richards and Irene Willis. New York: David McKay Co., 1976.

A guide to help adolescents deal with their parents' marital problems, their divorce, and its aftermath. (Ages 13 or 14 on up).

- (M) *Mushy Eggs.* Florence Adams. New York: G.P. Putnam's Sons, 1973 (32 pages).

David and Sam live in New York with their mother, who works, and their much-loved baby sitter, Fanny, while their father lives in New Jersey. Fanny retires and a new sitter comes, an upsetting situation at first. (Ages 3–8).

- (M) *A Friend Can Help.* Terry Berger. Milwaukee: Advanced Learning Concept and Children's Press, 1974 (32 pages).

Pictures reflect clearly the feelings of the characters. The girl in the story tells her best friend her feelings about her parents' divorce. (Ages 7–10)

• (M) *A Month of Sundays.* Rose Blue. New York: Franklin Watts, 1972 (272 pages, also Bantam paperback).

Jeff's parents divorce and he and his mother move to New York City. A friend, Matthew, and his adopted mother help, and Jeff begins to enjoy his new life. Helpful for children who feel that divorce and a different life style are the end of their world. (Ages 8–10)

• (B) *It's Not the End of the World.* Judy Blume. Scarsdale, N.Y.: Bradbury Press, 1972 (160 pages).

When her parents divorce, a sixth grader struggles to understand that sometimes people are unable to live together. (Ages 10–12)

• (B) *Where Is Daddy? The Story of a Divorce.* Beth Goff. Boston: Beacon Press, 1969 (32 pages).

A little girl who cannot understand her parents' divorce, blames herself, and fears her mother will not return when she goes to work. The story shows how her grandmother and mother help her. (Ages 4–7)

• (M) *I Know You, Al.* Constance C. Greene. New York: Viking Press, 1975 (128 pages).

Alexandra has a dual problem coping with her mother's boy friend and her father's upcoming wedding, necessitating a new dress and hair style. Another story revolves around feelings about being preadolescent. A friend describes the sequence of events in very believable terms. (Ages 11–14)

• (A) *Guy Lenny.* Harry Mazer. New York: Delacorte Press, 1971 (62 pages).

Twelve-year-old Guy has lived with his father for seven years, since his mother left for another man. Now his father wants to remarry, and at the same time his mother returns, insisting that Guy now live with her and her husband. Guy feels caught between them and betrayed by both; he behaves very badly. He has nonetheless developed an inner strength and independence. The story presents realistic dilemmas for families involved in divorce. (Ages 10–14)

• (A) *I, Trissy.* Norma Mazer. New York: Delacorte Press, 1971 (128 pages).

Trissy types her own story: she feels caught between her parents but blames her mother for the divorce. She behaves in a self-centered way, and she herself causes problems in the aftermath of the divorce. Her parents are understanding and she begins to build a more mature and responsible way of behaving. (Ages 10–13)

• (M) *A Father Like That.* Charlotte Zolotow. New York: Harper & Row, 1971 (24 pages).

A little boy tells his mother his dreams of the ideal father, as his own father "went away" before he was born. The story tells how he and his mother use this fantasy. (Ages 3–8)

• (A) *The Half Parent: Living With Other People's Children.* Brenda Maddox. New York: The New American Library, 1975 (204 pages).

About the parent by marriage, this is an exploration of the emotional and adjustment problems and rewards of living with other people's children.

• (A) *Remarriage.* Carmel Berman Reingold. New York: Harper & Row, 1976 (278 pages).

This was the first book to be published entirely on the subject of remarriage. Discusses such problems as the ex-spouse, stepchildren, in-laws, money, and making friends again.

• (A) *Living in Step.* Ruth Roosevelt and Jeanette Lofas. New York: Stein and Day, 1976 (248 pages).

The authors deal with the realities of remarriage and the complex family ties no one is experienced to handle.

## FILMS

The following is an annotated listing of mental health films. These films were chosen on the basis of personal experience, recommendations of colleagues, and reviews prepared by the Mental Health Materials Center. The reviewed films that are included were found to be either very good (***) or excellent (****) by the reviewing staff.

A fuller listing of mental health audio-visual aids can be found in *Current Audiovisuals for Mental Health Education,* 1979, edited by Jack Neher, Marquis Academic Media, 200 East Ohio Street, Chicago, Illinois 60611.

### Aggression and Violence

• *Childhood Aggression**** (31 min.,color,16 mm,1976).

This is a documentary about Tim, whose aggressive behavior upsets his family and causes problems at school. Referred to an experimental child psychotherapy research program, the family was carefully screened to determine whether they could manage the behavior modification approach of the project. These highly motivated parents quickly learned the necessary techniques and applied them to one specific behavior pattern that was particularly troublesome. Tim, too, played an active role in this program. When, after several months, Tim's aggressive behavior was diminished at home, the social learning techniques were tried with Tim's teachers and schoolmates. A most effective and absorbing film—and one that will be useful to spark discussion among professionals and trainees in child psychotherapy.
Distributor: Media Guild
P.O. Box 881
Solana Beach, California 92075

• *Battered Woman: Violence Behind Closed Doors**** (23 min., color, 16 mm, 1977).

Wife-beaters are more numerous than rapists. Family crisis calls make up about one-fourth of all calls to most police departments. Starting with these astonishing facts, this film goes on to examine some of the causes of domestic violence and to point out what should be done to help the victims. Behind the specific reasons given by the perpetrators (cold dinners, noisy children, supposed unfaithfulness) are some deep-seated social and psychological problems (alcoholism, sex role stereotyping, low esteem, inability to verbalize feelings, etc.). Although some police departments offer counseling services to abused women, there are still too few community services for them. In the film we hear from various men who have beaten their wives, from some battered women, from police officers who have intervened, and from a woman who runs a refuge for battered women. We thought the film would be fine for police training as well as for general information with community groups. There is an excellent discussion guide.

Distributor: J. Gary Mitchell Film Co.
163 Tunstead Avenue
San Anselmo, California 94960

- *Rape: A Preventive Inquiry**** (17½ min., color, 16 mm, 1976).

Four victims of rape attacks join several policemen in a discussion of ways to lessen chances of assault. Some convicted rapists also speak up but they sound brainwashed. Nevertheless, there is much good solid advice for girls and women in this film.

Distributor: J. Gary Mitchell Film Co.

- *Violent Youth***** (23 min., color, 16 mm, 1976).

With commendable honesty and objectivity, this film takes a hard look at what is now being done in the way of rehabilitating juveniles who have committed violent crimes and asks if we think society is preventing violence or provoking it. We meet three young offenders and we also hear from some professionals who have varying opinions on the efficacy of the offenders' treatment. No pat answers are provided by this realistic and troubling film but it raises some excellent points for discussion by parents as well as by workers in youth-serving community agencies.

Distributor: Harper & Row Media
10 E. 53rd St.
New York, New York 10022

## Death

• *To Die Today* (50 min. b/w, 16 mm, 1972).

Produced by the Canadian Broadcasting Corporation, this is the classic presentation of Dr. Elisabeth Kubler-Ross's theories, which have had such a humanizing effect on the care of the terminally ill. In it she describes the five emotional stages through which a dying patient passes: denial, anger, depression, preparatory grief, and acceptance. She emphasizes that awareness of these stages is essential in relating to the dying person.
Distributor: Filmakers Library, Inc.
133 East 58th Street, Suite 793A
New York, New York 10022

• *Death. Dying in a Hospital* (43 min. b/w, 16 mm, 1970).

This is an intensely personal study of 52-year-old Albro Pearsall dying of cancer at Calvary Hospital in New York. As the camera records the hospital routine, it reveals the response of staff, family, and patient to terminal illness.

The film will arouse many questions: Why is it so hard to communicate meaningfully with the dying patient? What are the patient's psychological defenses? What are the defenses of the caregivers?
Distributor: Filmakers Library, Inc.
133 East 58th Street, Suite 703 A
New York, New York 10022

## Divorce

• *Stepparenting: New Families, Old Ties**** (25 min., color, 16 mm, 1977).

Stepparents often feel they are "flying blind" in attempting to relate to their new families. Comparatively little has been written on this pervasive problem and there are no obvious sources of help. In this absorbing documentary, Henry and Marilyn Felt interview a number of articulate, thoughtful stepparents who found guidance by getting together with other stepparents in their community and by sharing problems and ideas. There's a good variety of adult personalities and situations in the film and the film

should be helpful to other stepparents who might want to start (or uncover) a similar group.
Distributor: Wombat Publications, Inc.
Little Lake, Glendale Rd.
P.O. Box 70
Ossining, New York 10562

- *Mothers After Divorce***** (20 min., color, 16 mm, 1977).

Four divorced women get together to talk about their problems and to share ideas for solving those problems. All have children of high school age and all have had to go back to work.. Furthermore, all are highly articulate and quite moving as they describe their feelings about their former and their present lives. We also see these women at home with their families or functioning at their jobs so the film is not just talking heads. We thought it would make an excellent discussion starter for single-parent groups as well as for the professionals who counsel them. Beyond that, the film would be pertinent for college classes in marriage and family life. It could even be used with the general public to stimulate discussion on life styles. This is an unusually good film that will be welcomed by persons who use films in staff training or community education.
Distributor: Polymorph Films
331 Newbury St.
Boston, Massachusetts 02115

**Drug and Sex Education**

- *Balancing Head and Heart***** (series of seven half-hour video tapes, b/w, 1974).

Subtitled "Sensible Ideas for the Prevention of Drug and Alcohol Abuse," this new series of videotapes is indeed sensible and full of ideas. Designed for use with program planners, teachers, parents, and others concerned with drug and alcohol education programs in the schools, this series takes an in-depth look at eleven strategies now being employed in American schools (e.g., The Magic Circle, School Without Failure, Cross-Age Tutoring, Parent Effectiveness Training). Used individually or as a series, these tapes can be the basis of teacher-training workshops and seminars.
Distributor: Prevention Materials Institute
P.O. Box 152
Lafayette, California 94549

• *Growing Up Young* (22 min., color, sound, 16 mm, Super-8 mm, Video-Cassettes).

Made especially for teen-aged audiences, this film explores the special problems of adolescent sexuality and the need for friendship and approval that is the context within which decisions about sex are made.
Distributor: Perennial Education, Inc.
477 Roger Williams
P.O. Box 885 Ravinia
Highland Park, Illinois 60035

**Learning Disabilities and Childhood Autism**

• *The I.Q. Myth***** (51 min., color, 16 mm, 1976).

Originally shown on CBS television, this documentary provides an excellent review of the IQ concept and its problems. Various educational and psychological luminaries (Jerome Kagan of Harvard is the most interesting, but they are all good) testify against the IQ test, showing that it really works only with upper- or middle-class children and even then reveals little but an aptitude for school work. The second part illustrates how IQ tests have been used to label children in ways that seriously affect their future lives. This absorbing film should be seen by all parents of school-age children, but its best use would probably be with teachers or teachers-in-training—to help them sort out the facts from the myths surrounding "IQ."
Distributor: Carousel Films
1501 Broadway
New York, New York 10036

• *If A Boy Can't Learn**** (28 min., color, 16 mm, 1976).

Cowboy Mike, aged 17, enters high school a hard-core nonreader, unable to do math and antagonistic to discipline. Deep down, however, Mike has a heart of gold. A concerned teacher refers him to a learning disability center, where Mike gets a battery of tests. (There's an excellent sequence in which a psychologist explains to Mike's parents that their son has difficulty in understanding what he hears.) The tests indicate a change in teaching methods for Mike and the next step is to get the faculty to devise strategies. Role playing is one technique used to get Mike interested and involved in his studies. The result is a marked change in Mike's attitude. Perhaps the best thing about

the film is the footage devoted to the diagnostic process and subsequent alteration of teaching methods. There are many ideas here for teachers as well as guidance personnel. The film should also be seen by parents as well as students of psychology.
Distributor: Lawren Productions, Inc.
P.O. Box 666
Mendocino, California 95460

• *More Than Hugs and Kisses* (23 min., color, 16 mm, 1980).

Filmed in a class of three-to-seven-year olds at the Jowonio School in Syracuse, N.Y., this film follows the typical school day, showing reading and arithmetic, fun and conflict. What is unusual is the special attention the teacher pays to the personal and interpersonal needs of the children.

Observing each child individually, Ms. Brogan determines personal psychoeducational goals. Then, through sequential activities and spontaneous intervention when called for, she helps her students improve their communication skills and their behavior. This method works for both the typical children as well as the special children, whose problems include autism, retardation, and emotional disturbance.
Produced by: Grania Gurievitch, Togg Films
Filmakers Library, Inc.
133 East 58th St., Suite 703A
New York, New York 10022

• *The Edge of Awareness**** (27 min., color, 16 mm, 1975).

This film shows an absorbing visit to Boston's Language and Cognitive Development Center, where a number of interesting new techniques are employed to help autistic and aphasic children. Most of the film is devoted to a demonstration of a unique obstacle course that forces the child to employ all his or her body skills. The film also shows how parents can acquire these techniques to teach survival skills to their children. A handsome and useful training film for staff members of schools and clinics serving autistic children.
Distributor: Cognitive Development Designs, Inc.
25 Huntington Ave.
Boston, Massachusetts 02116

- *A Boy Named Terry Egan**** (2 parts: 30 min. each, b/w, color, 16 mm, 1973).

This film covers virtually every aspect of childhood autism, including the thorny problem of community hostility to treatment facilities. We see Terry (age 9) at home with parents and siblings and in a special school. Emphasis is on helping Terry get into public schools, avoiding hospitalization. We are shown the interesting technique of "intrusion time," getting the autistic child to respond to stimuli, which is taught to his parents by the treatment center's staff. The film is useful for community education programs as well as staff training or recruitment programs.
Distributor: Carousel Films, Inc.
1501 Broadway
New York, New York 10036

**Stress**

- *Four Women: Breast Cancer***** (55 min., color, 16 mm, 1979).

This film is the personal story of four women who underwent the operation most feared by women, mastectomy. With unflinching honesty it explores the physical and psychological effects of the surgery. Three of the women are married with young children. They and their husbands speak about their fears and uncertainties and the kind of adjustments they had to make after hospitalization. One woman describes her experience with breast reconstruction.

The content of the film makes it useful for professionals who work with cancer patients and for patient education programs.
Produced by: Canadian Broadcasting Corporation
Filmakers Library, Inc.
133 East 58th St., Suite 703A
New York, New York 10022

- *Stress Training for Teachers**** (three 16-min., color, 16 mm films, 1976).

These three brief films are intended for use primarily in teacher training. "The Crunch" deals with highly disruptive class behavior. "Black Is the Color" deals with a white teacher's fear of black students. "Crossing the Line" concerns a well-meaning teacher's interference in a student's life. The

format is interesting: each film has a basic story line that is interrupted with comments from teachers and students. Our reviewers thought the stories a bit melodramatic (though some thought they were not exaggerated) but useful in the long run as discussion material for junior and senior high school teacher training.
Distributor: Film Modules
496 Deer Park Ave.
Babylon, New York 11702

• *Self-Management of Behavior**** (33 min., color, 16 mm, 1976).

Another behavior modification film, but this one has commentary by B. F. Skinner, who says, among other provocative things, "You control yourself by controlling the environment." Two cases of "unmanageable" boys are presented and we are shown the techniques employed by therapists and parents in helping the boys learn self-control. To the basic idea of giving tangible rewards for good behavior is added the concept of self-regulation: the child keeps his own records of his progress. Well-made and consistently interesting, but probably chiefly for professionals or students in child therapy.
Distributor: Media Guild
P.O. Box 881
Solana Beach, California 92075

• *Psychotherapy**** (25 min., color, 16 mm, 1977).

Several case histories are acted out to explain what goes on in psychotherapy. First we see an initial interview in which the psychiatrist describes to the patient what he plans to do. One of his goals is to provide a safe relationship, to build a sense of mutual agreement with both patient and therapist working together. The next sequence demonstrates "working through" and transference, while the final episode shows a patient trying out new patterns of behavior and preparing to terminate therapy. The narrator tells us that there are many different kinds of therapy but all have the same objective: "to help the patient get in touch with the reservoir of motivation that lies outside his or her awareness." We thought it well done, if somewhat oversimplified, but useful as an introduction to psychotherapy for students, employees of mental health treatment facilities, and the general public.
Distributor: Davidson Films
163 Tunsted Ave.
San Anselmo, California 94960

- *One Man's Madness**** (31 min., color, 16 mm, 1975).

In this British documentary, a writer describes his struggles to cope with manic-depressive episodes. We also hear from his wife, who says "There's a boring side to coping with mental illness," and his psychiatrist, who says he can treat some of the symptoms but still doesn't know what causes this man's illness. Although there are too many shots of the protagonist walking toward the camera as he talks to us, the film does a good job of showing the effect of mental illness upon a family. There are also interesting scenes of the patient in the hospital during one of his periods of depression. Possibly the best thing about this film is that it humanizes mental illness, making this one man's illness very real to the viewers.
Distributor: Time-Life Multimedia
100 Eisenhower Dr.
Paramus, New Jersey 07652

## SUMMARY

Mental health practitioners are often called upon to educate as well as to heal. Books, pamphlets, and movies are also helpful aids when presenting public talks. This chapter has provided an annotated bibliography on a multitude of mental health and child development books, pamphlets, and movies.

Chapter 9

# Chemotherapy

# 9

Mental health clinicians, whether medical or nonmedical, whether they practice in the public or private sector, are knowledgeable in the art and science of healing. They have their "pet" theories and an abundance of techniques and therapeutic strategies that provide direction to their psychotherapeutic encounters with patients. However, by contrast, most independent practitioners' fund of general information regarding chemotherapy is lacking. The purpose of this chapter is to remedy that situation.

Chemotherapy plays an important role in the treatment of mentally and emotionally disturbed individuals. The serious use of psychotropic drugs as a treatment strategy has made it possible for the community to care for the acutely ill, and has greatly facilitated their adaptability to noninstitutionalized living. During the 1950s and 1960s, when psychotropic drugs were introduced as "psychiatry's answer to penicillin," nonmedically oriented practitioners and their medically oriented colleagues became polarized around whether the inappropriate thoughts, feelings, and actions of disturbed people were based on functional (nonchemical) or structural (chemical) causes. Should the treatment focus on unconscious dreams and schemes or on genes and amines?

Today the value of drugs in the treatment of emotionally disturbed adults and children cannot be denied. More and more nonmedically oriented practitioners find themselves coming into contact with patients who are either taking medication, might benefit from medication, or themselves raise issues regarding medication. This chapter will provide some familiarity with the use of drug therapy.

Numerous classifications have been designed to organize the multiple drugs and their uses: i.e., tranquilizers, sedatives, neuroleptic psyche inhibitors. A nomenclature that is based on clinical usage is the most helpful. Drugs used for treating anxiety should be thought of as antianxiety drugs, those for mental depression as antidepressants, and those used for treating psychotics and schizophrenics as antipsychotic drugs.

When considering medication for use with children, it is more helpful to consider target symptoms rather than diagnostic categories or behavior disorders.

## ADULTS

Choca (1980) has summarized the major uses of psychotropic drugs. Tables 9–1 to 9–4, and the discussion of possible side effects, are reproduced with his permission.

**Table 9–1** Anti-Anxiety Drugs

*Actions:*

1. Reduction of anxieties or tensions for periods of acute stress
2. Decrease of motor activity
3. Relaxation of muscles
4. Detoxification of alcohol or drug-addicted patients

*Side Effects:*

1. Lethargy, drowsiness, dizziness or disorientation
2. Lack of coordination
3. Skin rashes
4. Increased sensitivity to alcohol
5. Tendency towards habit formation
6. Menstrual irregularities
7. Jaundice
8. Bone marrow suppression

*Contraindications:*

1. Pregnancy
2. Children under six
3. Hazardous occupation that requires alertness

*Delay:* One hour

| Drug Type | Trade Name | Generic Name | Specific Actions | Dosage (mg) |
|---|---|---|---|---|
| Benzodiazepines | Librium | Chlordiazepoxide | Safer in case of OD | 15-300 |
| | Valium | Diazepam | | 5-60 |
| | Serax | Oxezepam | | 30-120 |
| Carbamates | Equanil | Meprobamate | Unsafe and addictive | 400-1600 |
| | Miltown | " | | |
| Diphenylmethane | Atarax | Hydroxyzine | | 75-400 |
| | Vistaril | " | | " |

## **Table 9–2** Anti-Psychotic Drugs

*Actions:*

1. Orders the thought process
2. Decreases motor activity
3. Reduces delusions and hallucinations
4. Reduces tension and anxieties

*Side Effects:*

1. Extrapyramidal symptoms (see text for description)
2. Lack of coordination, difficulty and pain in movement
3. Tardive dyskinesia (see text)
4. Dizziness, drowsiness, weakness, confusion or stupor
5. Dryness of mouth and throat
6. Nasal congestion
7. Nausea, vomiting, constipation or diarrhea
8. Urinary disturbance
9. Blurred vision
10. Drop of blood pressure when standing up, tachycardia
11. Inhibition of ejaculation (especially Mellaril)
12. Menstrual irregularities
13. Skin oversensitivity to sun, skin rashes
14. Lowering of seizure threshold, convulsions
15. Jaundice
16. Weight gain

*Contraindications:*

1. Previous sensitivity
2. Comatose states, brain damage
3. Previous intake of large amounts of alcohol, barbiturates or narcotics
4. Hazardous occupation that requires alertness

*Delay:* Several Days

| Drug Type | Trade Name | Generic Name | Specific Action | Dosage (mg) |
|---|---|---|---|---|
| Aliphatic | Thorazine | Chlorpromazine | Strong sedative effect | 50-1000 |
| Piperazine | Stelazine | Trifluoperazine | 1. Low sedative effect | 5-30 |
| | Trilafon | Perphenazine | | 12-64 |
| | Prolixon | Fluphenazine | 2. Prolixin Decanoate is long-acting, | 1-20 |
| | Repoise | Butaperazine | injectable form | 15-100 |
| | Compazine | Prochlorperazine | 3. Prone to side effect #1 | 10-40 |
| Piperidine | Quide | Piperacetazine | Not prone to side effect #1, #3 | 10-160 |
| | Serentil | Mesoridazine | | 50-400 |
| | Mellaril | Thioridazine | | 50-800 |

*(continues)*

**Table 9–2** continued

| Drug Type | Trade Name | Generic Name | Specific Action | Dosage (mg) |
|---|---|---|---|---|
| Butyrophenones | Haldol | Haloperidol | 1. Prone to side effect #1 | 2-100 |
| | | | 2. Low sedative effect | |
| Thioxanthenes | Taractan<br>Navane | Chlorprothixene<br>Thiothixene | | 25-600<br>5-30 |
| Indolone | Mobane | Molindone | Low sedative effect | 25-400 |
| Dibenzoxazepine | Loxitane | Loxapine | 1. Strong sedative effect<br>2. Marked side effect #1, #14 | 25-400<br>20-100 |
| Phenothiazine and Tricyclic | Triavil<br>Etrafon | Perphenazine and Amitriptyline | Combination anti-psychotic and anti-depressant | |

**Table 9–3** Anti-Depressant Drugs

*Actions:*

1. Mood elevation
2. Reduction of psychomotor retardation
3. Increase of motivation and optimism

*Side Effects:*

1. Extrapyramidal symptoms (see text for description)
2. Lack of coordination, difficulty and pain in movement
3. Dizziness, drowsiness, weakness, confusion or stupor
4. Dryness of mouth and throat
5. Nausea, vomiting, constipation or diarrhea
6. Urinary disturbance
7. Blurred vision
8. Drop in blood pressure when standing up
9. Tachycardia (rapid heart rate), palpitations
10. Lowering of seizure threshold, convulsions
11. Accelerated psycho-motor activity
12. Activation of psychotic symptoms like hallucinations and delusions
13. Insomnia
14. Weight gain or loss
15. Perspiration

*Contraindications:*

1. Prostatic hypertrophy (with tricyclics)
2. Glaucoma (with tricyclics)
3. Recent myocardial infarction
4. Arrhythmia

*Delay:* Two to four weeks

**Table 9–3** continued

| Drug Type | Trade Name | Generic Name | Specific Action | Dosage (mg) |
|---|---|---|---|---|
| Tricyclics | Elavil | Amitriptyline | | 50-225 |
| | Norpramine | Desipramine | | 75-200 |
| | Tofranil | Imipramine | | 50-225 |
| | Aventyl | Nortriptyline | | 20-100 |
| | Vivactyl | Protriptyline | | 10-60 |
| | Sinequan | Doxepin HCl | | 40-200 |
| MAO Inhibitors | Marplan | Isocarboxazid | Excessive Toxicity | 10-50 |
| | Nardil | Phenelzine | Excessive Toxicity | 15-75 |
| | Parnate | Tranylcyptomine | Excessive Toxicity | 10-30 |

**Table 9–4** Lithium Carbonate

*Actions:* Treatment of Manic Depressive Illness

1. Decrease of elation and acceleration of psychomotor activity to manic states
2. Increase of optimism, motivation and psychomotor activity in depressed states

*Side Effects:*

1. Nausea, vomiting, diarrhea or abdominal pain
2. Muscular weakness
3. Sluggish or dazed feeling
4. Thirst and excessive urination
5. Fine hand tremor

Intoxication produces drowsiness, tremors, slurred speech, convulsions and coma

*Contraindications:*

1. Thyroid deficiency
2. Renal deficiency
3. Liver deficiency
4. Cardiovascular disease
5. Patients on diuretics

*Delay:* One to three weeks

| Trade Name | Generic Name | Specifications | Dosage (mg) |
|---|---|---|---|
| Lithonate | Lithium Carbonate | Must reach blood levels of 0.8 to 1.2 milliequivalents per liter for therapeutic effect. Toxic above 2.0 Eq/li | 300-2500 |
| Liphane | | | |
| Lithotabs | | | |
| Eskalith | | | |

Most of the possible side effects are seldom seen. An exception to this rule, however, are the *extrapyramidal* symptoms frequently seen with the use of anti-psychotic or tricyclic antidepressants. These side effects may be suppressed with the use of antiparkinsonian agents. The extrapyramidal symptoms may include:

- Akathisia or restlessness with inability to sleep, a compulsion to walk and an inability to be still.
- Dyskinesias and dystonias which may include jerking or spastic movements, upward deviation of the eyes, spasms of the neck and in severe cases, spasms of the mouth and pharynx with inability to speak or swallow.
- Parkinsonian Syndrome or Parkinsonism which includes tremors, muscular rigidity of limbs and face (mask-like facies) and slowness or scarcity of movements with lack of associated movements such as arm swing.

The extrapyramidal effects tend to disappear after a period of time. As a result, the usual technique is to add the antiparkinsonian drug when the symptoms appear and plan to reduce and discontinue this medication four months thereafter. At that point the symptoms may not reappear, even when the individual continues to take the psychotropic drug. This procedure encourages discontinuing medications that the patient no longer needs.

About 5% of the patients who take antipsychotic medications for some period of time develop *tardive dyskinesia.* This syndrome is characterized by a sucking-like puckering of the lips; chewing, licking or pursing movements of the tongue or mouth; or choreiform movements of the extremities. Tardive dyskinesia is irreversible in most cases and there is no known treatment. If detected, the drug should be discontinued if at all possible. If the risk of relapse is too great, Mellaril, which is the least likely to produce this disorder, may be used after informed consent has been obtained.

## CHILDREN

In contrast to adult patients, the efficacy of psychotropic drugs as a treatment agent has not been scientifically demonstrated or as widely adapted by mental health personnel who work with children and adolescents (Gittelman-Klein, 1975; Halpern & Kissel, 1976; Campbell & Small, 1980). The successful use of chemotherapy with the minimal brain dysfunction child has stimulated wider use and acceptance of drugs as a treatment agency in children. While it is recognized that drugs will not alter parents' attitudes, change children's intelligence, or create learning, they can help a child to become more accessible to environmental manipulations such as special educational programs. Extensive reviews of the use and effectiveness of drug therapy with children can be found in Campbell and Small (1978) and Halpern and Kissel (1976).

Eisenberg (1971) outlined several principles of drug therapy in child psychiatry. He considered the use of medication as only a component part of a total treatment program for the disturbed child. In each case the potential risks of taking chemicals into the body must be weighed against the anticipated benefits and costs to the individual if the drug is not given. Symptomatic relief need not be disparaged if it improves a child's functioning.

In general, the following guidelines are essential when considering the strategy of utilizing chemotherapy techniques:

- Drugs should be used only if there are firm indications for them.
- An old drug, one that has been available for a time, is better than a new one, unless the latter's superiority has been proved.
- Drugs should be used at the lowest effective dosage and no longer than necessary.
- The degree of morbidity from both use or nonuse of the drug should be taken into account in determining the cost to the well-being of the child.

The following discussion regarding the use of drugs in children for ameliorating the distressing effects of specific symptoms is based on a portion of previously published work of Halpern and Kissel (1976) and is reprinted with the permission of the publisher.

Pharmacologic agents have been found for only a few target symptoms and functions. Of these, the following list represents the most common difficulties that are usually sensitive to specific medication:

1. Hyperkinesis
2. Enuresis
3. Encopresis
4. Sleep disorders
5. Depression
6. Mania
7. Anorexia
8. Obesity
9. Tics
10. Phobias
11. Learning problems

### Hyperkinesis

Nearly forty years ago Bradley (1937) described the use of amphetamine (Benzedrine-R), a stimulant drug, in the treatment of behavior disorders of children. Shortly thereafter dextroamphetamine (Dexedrine-R) was found to be even more effective (Bradley, 1950). By 1953 Ginn and Hohman reported that excessive restlessness was most responsive to dextroamphetamine. Although a variety of symptoms such as short attention span, impulsiveness, temper outbursts, poor concentration, and quarrelsomeness improved concomitantly, it was chiefly the driven motor behavior that was often dramatically turned off by this drug and thus the drug came to be thought of as a specific treatment modality for the hyperkinetic syndrome (Eisenberg et al., 1963; Weiss et al., 1971a,b). Because approximately four in every hundred grade school children are believed to be hyperkinetic (Millichap, 1968), the importance of the drug for classroom management and indirectly for improving academic performance was not lost on educators (Freeman, 1966). Public outcry about the potential for political abuse and social control was not far behind (Grinspoon & Singer, 1973).

Stimulant drugs are considered a proper modality of treatment for hyperkinetic children if integrated into a total treatment program that addresses itself to the child in his or her situation rather than to solely symptomatic activity (Eisenberg, 1971; 1972). Since the syndrome may encompass a variety of problems stemming from diverse causes, overreliance on one drug seems hardly realistic (Fish, 1971). Moreover, the differential effects of these drugs on aspects of behavior have yet to be thoroughly explored (Arnold et al., 1973).

A stimulant of a different chemical structure, methylphenidate (Ritalin), has virtually supplanted the amphetamines (Campbell et al., 1971; Schleifer et al., 1975), because it has a comparable effect without being invested with the socially stigmatizing quality of "speed." Although claims have been made for fewer side effects with methylphenidate, there is some doubt about this earlier position. Like dextroamphetamine, it tends to cause insomnia, depressed appetite, and reduced physical growth (Safer et al., 1972; Safer & Allen, 1973), although the last finding has been refuted in a retrospective study of adolescents (Beck et al., 1975). Dextroamphetamine is more likely to be utilized for hyperkinetic preschoolers because a liquid preparation is available, whereas no such form is available for methylphenidate. A third central nervous system stimulant, structurally different from the aforementioned two drugs, is pemoline (Cylert-R), which can be administered on a once-daily dosage regimen. In addition to improving gross motor behavior, some positive effects on cognitive and perceptual functions have also been recorded (Conners et al., 1972; Page et al., 1974). Caffeine in the form of well-brewed coffee has had good results for one practitioner (Schnackenberg, 1973).

One of the major concerns about the introduction of stimulants in the treatment of hyperactive children has centered about the danger of habituation and later drug abuse (Koupernick, 1972). All evidence over a 30-year period strongly suggests the absence of such proclivity in treated children while medicated and during several years of post-treatment observation (Beck et al., 1975; Laufer, 1971a; 1971b).

*Case A*

The mother of two children applied for service on the advice of her son's nursery school teacher and pediatrician because the youngster did not get along with other children. For example, he would repeatedly ride his tricycle rough shod through a group of children and seemed not to learn from the negative attention he received for this behavior. Those who observed him in the nursery and in the neighborhood believed that he liked getting into scraps. He took his parents' full attention to the point that they felt neglectful of an 11-year-old daughter who was 7 years his senior.

From birth on the boy was considered to be a much more difficult child than the sister had been. As a baby he had been fretful, colicky, and restless in the night. The parents believed that he had never slept through a night as they would often hear him get up and go to the bathroom, or drink water, or simply busy himself in his bedroom when he was expected to be asleep. Television viewing had to be curtailed since he would become too excited with certain programs. His hyperactivity during the day was expressed in terms of "wildness" when he was unable to stop himself from running around and when his excitement interfered with his awareness of others. At age one he had been given phenobarbital for his irritability, but this medication had caused a paradoxic increase in wakefulness and in discomfort.

When the child was seen clinically in the office there was no sign that would lead one to suspect that he was hyperactive, least of all that he was prone to lose self-control. However, when he was observed in an open group setting or in the waiting room his driven behavior became quickly evident. The child was treated with methylphenidate (Ritalin), 20 mg being the most effective daily dose. When he entered the first grade, he was teased by other children about taking a pill at noon so that the medication was changed to a long-acting form of dextroamphetamine 10 mg (Dexedrine Spansule-R).

With this regimen, he continued his improved behavior in school, where he was sufficiently attentive and calm to benefit from the teacher's instructions. During vacations, the parents were supported in their desire to have the boy take a drug holiday. On follow-up visits the child indicated that he felt better about himself since he was on medication. One side effect, the fact that he cried more easily, had initially troubled the parents since they were not accustomed to his ever being weepy.

*Case B*

The recently divorced mother of three girls was referred for help by the school social worker in order to check out what could be done for the oldest child, who was about to repeat kindergarten. This girl was described as immature and hyperkinetic. Her birth weight had been somewhat over four pounds. Because the mother believed her to have suffered most from the breakup of the family, she requested psychotherapy for this daughter and herself.

On being seen, the girl exhibited driven behavior and pressured speech. It was difficult to sort out the situational or reactive factors from an endogenous problem with hyperkinesis. The decision was made to at least try stimulant medication while starting a course of play therapy for the child and collateral counseling for the mother. Ritalin, 10 mg twice daily, had an immediate positive effect on the outward manifestations of overactivity, although there was good reason to continue in treatment with the child, who tended to be negativistic, demanding, and manipulative. After ten months of weekly collateral meetings, the girl was thought to be sufficiently improved so that play therapy was discontinued. However, she remained on her medication for another two years while she matured. One year after the medication was stopped, she was reported to be making an adequate school adjustment.

The dosage schedule for these medications must be titrated to a child's idiosyncratic response. Some children show a clear-cut drop in their driven behavior with low dosages, while others require much higher amounts before there is a notable improvement. Sometimes, one of the stimulants works better than the other so that each should be considered as a potential alternative in case of poor response or of undesirable side effects.

A suggested dosage schedule for three of these drugs is given below. Ordinarily a starting dose of dextroamphetamine is 2.5 mg on arising and after lunch for preschoolers, while for older children 5 mg twice daily or 5–10 mg of methylphenidate morning and noon is recommended.

| | Initial mg/kg body weight/per day |
|---|---|
| Dextroamphetamine | 0.25 |
| Methylphenidate | 0.25 |
| Pemoline | 0.50 |

| | Optimum mg/kg body weight/per day |
|---|---|
| Dextroamphetamine | 1.00 |
| Methylphenidate | 2.00 |
| Pemoline | 4.00 |

These amounts may be increased until the desired improvement occurs or until side effects intrude. Furthermore, the dosage may have to be adjusted over time in keeping with the maturational changes of the child. Vacation periods are looked upon as good opportunities for cutting back or withholding medication. This is to see if the requirements for its use still exist and to obviate potentially deleterious consequences of chronic drug use such as those recorded on appetite and rate of physical growth (Safer et al., 1972). Idiosyncratic side effects have been reported (Mattson & Calverley, 1968) but are not common (Conners, 1972).

When other methods fail, the multifaceted antidepressant imipramine (Tofranil), although less efficient in the amelioration of hyperactivity than the stimulants, is thought to have some applicability in the management of this problem (Rapoport, 1965; Quinn & Rapoport, 1975). However, in the desirable dosages it may precipitate major seizures in children who have evidence of organic brain disease but who are without a history of convulsions (Brown et al., 1974). In susceptible patients in whom seizures intervene with stimulants or antidepressants, a lowering of the dosage and supplemental anticonvulsants should be used (Millichap, 1968).

## Enuresis

Nocturnal enuresis or automatic bedwetting while asleep probably affects two to three million children in the United States (Muellner, 1960). Most instances stem from physiologically determined immaturity of bladder capacity and control, although psychological factors occasionally may be contributory to this symptom formation. In any event, it is a distressing problem to the child and as often to his or her parents. The number of drugs and devices deployed in its remediation is a sign of the anxious effort devoted to its management. In 1960, McLean reported that imipramine (Tofranil) benefited bedwetters, and since then a host of articles have appeared attesting its efficacy in this respect (Margolis, 1962; Munster et al., 1961; Poussaint & Ditman, 1965). To decrease nocturnal enuresis in children under twelve years of age, 25–50 mg of imipramine are given at bedtime for up to two months, when it is withdrawn. The dose may be increased to 75 mg in children over twelve years of age. At the end of this program many children have been "trained" to be dry. Some children remain poor responders or eventually escape the drug's restraint. The precise action is not known but it is believed that the anticholinergic effect of the drug brings about an increased capacity of the bladder to hold urine and that its stimulant effect on the central nervous system makes the individual more aware of a full bladder. Side reactions may include dryness of the mouth and constipation as well as greater aggressiveness (Tec, 1963) and electrocardiographic changes (Martin & Zang, 1975).

*Case C*

An eight-year-old boy, the middle of three children, wet his bed nightly. Medical investigation had ruled out a clear-cut organic basis for the enuresis. The middle-class parents, whose two daughters were dry at night, had tried all kinds of methods to help their son with this problem, although he was not visibly upset by it. He was an alert, active child who had friends, did well in school, and seemed rather fastidious in his personal grooming. It had been noted that he was dry on the one occasion when he slept at a friend's house.

Using this pretext the parents came for help because they believed that emotional reasons only could explain the phenomenon of selective bedwetting. When the therapist spoke with the boy, he learned that the youngster had been worried about embarrassing himself by wetting and had tried not to sleep. In all likelihood, he did not reach the deeper sleep stages during which automatic voiding usually occurs.

A trial of imipramine (Tofranil) 25 mg at bedtime served to eliminate the wetting for two nights only. The dosage was increased to 50 mg nightly with excellent control of the symptom. After two weeks the dosage was reduced and then withdrawn. When wetting recurred within a few days, the medication was again administered at the higher dosage for one month before being again withdrawn. The enuresis did not recur.

**Encopresis**

Children who have a problem with fecal soiling on a functional basis suffer even more as they often become social pariahs and a source of chagrin or embarrassment to their parents. At one time this symptom was viewed as a serious sign of underlying conflict between mother and child, who were thought to be locked into a hostile-dependent relationship (Bellman, 1966; Call et al, 1963). This explanation may well have mistaken the emotional and traumatic consequence of soiling for its cause. Berg and Jones (1964) distinguished several types of retentive and nonretentive encopresis, for which they outlined appropriate treatment plans, including therapy with the family and oral laxatives such as senna (Senokot-R) for the child. Abrahams (1963) reported one child's encopresis being relieved by imipramine

(Tofranil). More recently, good results have been reported for the nonretentive type with imipramine, which seems to be contraindicated in the retentive type of encopresis (Gavanski, 1971).

When retentive constipation and secondary leakage pose a problem, training or retraining of the bowels may remove the cause. An angry or frightened child or one phobic of toilets may, in withholding feces, form an impacted mass and secondarily an atonic sigmoid colon. Defecation quickly threatens to become a painful experience that the child avoids at all cost. The incontinence starts when fecal leakage occurs around the impaction. By returning control over his or her bowels to the child, there is good likelihood that routine toileting will be resumed. Rather than utilizing oral laxatives, the effect over which the child would have no control, using a quick-acting rectal suppository will empty the bowels 15–30 minutes after insertion so that evacuation can be arranged under predetermined conditions. Usually the child is directed to sit on the commode after this procedure and is rewarded with a small gift on successful evacuation into the toilet. A safe substance for this purpose is a bisacodyl (Dulcolax-R) suppository of 10 mg, which is inserted once daily for three successive days before beginning a trial of two days without medication to see whether the child will go to the bathroom spontaneously. Rewarding the child during the suppository-free period is continued, contingent on the successful moving of stool into the toilet, until the bowel habit is well established. Should retention of stool recur, a repetition of this treatment is required. Of course, associated interpersonal or phobic difficulties that might have given rise to the problem in the first place need to be attended to concurrently through appropriate psychotherapy or family counseling.

## Sleep Disorders

Children may undergo periods of insomnia at different stages, which may be puzzling and disturbing. On the whole, hypnotics and sedatives are to be avoided except for brief intervals when relief needs to be offered to the child and to the parent. Chloral hydrate (Notec-R) and diphenhydramine (Benadryl) are commonly employed for this response. Some hyperactive children do well with a bedtime dose of their stimulant medication as they may experience a rebound effect after the daytime medication has worn off (Laufer, 1971b).

Sleep walking or somnambulism is estimated to afflict 15 percent of all children between five and twelve years of age at least once. It is related to the shifting sleep stages from "nonrapid eye movement" (NREM) to "rapid eye movement" (REM) sleep in the neurologically immature child. A related phenomenon is pavor nocturnus, or night terrors, whereby a child is aroused into a panic state while remaining asleep. No specific psychological etiology has been demonstrated. Although these phenomena, really disorders of arousal, usually disappear spontaneously with age, the use of diazepam (Valium) at bedtime has been helpful in controlling them (Anders & Weinstein, 1972).

Narcolepsy, or involuntary dropping off into sleep, usually starts in childhood and is very responsive to central nervous stimulants, which are considered symptomatic treatment for the disorder. Methylphenidate (Ritalin) 10–20 mg three times per day before meals is preferred to dextroamphetamine (Dexedrine) or methamphetamine (Desoxyn-R) since it is reported to have fewer side effects (Yoss & Daly, 1960).

### Depression

Affective disorders in childhood are generally masked by behavioral problems. Presumably, if depressive states of childhood are to be better delineated, the discovery of biochemical correlates would prove most helpful in their identification (Cytryn et al., 1974) since antidepressant drugs like imipramine (Tofranil) can be most effective (Frommer, 1967). Their use in adolescents is no different from that of adults.

### Mania

There is some evidence that mood disorders with manic or cyclic stages occur before adolescence (Feinstein & Wolpert, 1973). Lithium carbonate (Eskalith-R, Lithane-R, Lithonate-R) is the drug of choice for abatement and prevention of mania (Annell, 1969). Blood serum levels must be monitored between 0.5–1.5 mEq/1, which is considered the effective range short of toxicity. Campbell et al. (1972a) noted that a child's autoaggressive and explosive behavior ceased on lithium when all other methods failed.

#### *Case D*

A sixteen-year-old high school student, the son of a lawyer, dropped out of school in order to travel. When he was arrested for possession of marijuana, he appeared unusually "high." At first his behavior was looked upon as drug related, but when the youth persisted in advertising himself fervently as mankind's savior, he was brought to psychiatric attention.

On examination he was hypomanic, suspicious of all authority other than his own, and expansive about his powers of understanding people. The history revealed a similar episode two years previous when the youth had run away from home for the first time after rejecting the control of home and school. After a two-month absence, during which he had lived a marginal existence in a hippie community, he became depressed and returned home. He looked upon this excursion as a defeat and awaited the magical age of sixteen to strike out again independently.

The diagnosis of a mood disorder of the manic-depressive type was entertained and lithium carbonate prescribed to attenuate the manic behavior. Within days after this regimen was instituted, he became less pressured in speech and action, dropped his allusions to being a spiritual power, and began to make more realistic plans for himself. He returned to school and graduated one year after his classmates while remaining on a daily maintenance dose of 600 mg lithium and requiring only periodic follow-up visits.

### Anorexia

A condition characterized by food aversion and associated loss of weight of serious proportions has come in for much clinical attention as a result of its refractoriness to treatment. All manner of regimens and therapies have been advanced, each reaching some patients in positive ways but clearly not reversing the process for all. What works in some seems anathema to others. A treatment approach that uses multiple modalities in keeping with the dynamics of the patient offers most hope (Tolstrup, 1975). Some clinicians look upon food as something that can be prescribed like medicine. The patient's weight is determined daily, and only evidenced weight gains lead to the granting of desirable privileges (Galdston, 1974). Neuroleptics of the phenothiazine group such as chlorpromazine (Thorazine-R) have been recommended to promote appetite (Dally & Sargant, 1966).

### Obesity

Lorber (1966) recommends that drug therapy be used with utmost restraint for exogenously overweight children. In grossly obese children, only when all previous dietary treatment has not been adhered to, a trial of anorectic drugs is indicated. Even then, long-term results are poor unless the whole family can also be treated, sometimes aided and abetted by high incentive group effort or mutual support. Unlike the case in adults, the use of a slow release amphetamine (Dexedrine Spansule) or prolonged action phenmetrazine hydrochloride (Preludin-R) in children affords short-term weight loss without causing restlessness, excitability, habit formation, or withdrawal symptoms.

### Involuntary Tics and Other Movements

A syndrome of involuntary tics and utterances that may be coprolalic was first described in 1885 by Gilles de la Tourette. Its onset occurs usually between the second and sixteenth year, more often in boys, and may persist for months or years. An organic attribute of unknown etiology contributes to its unfolding, but psychological factors may also influence its expression (Stevens & Blachly, 1966). In its major form the manifestations of the syndrome have a devastating impact on the child's social adjustment and academic life (Rosenthal et al., 1975). Triflupromazine (Vesprin ), thioridazine (Mellaril), diazepam (Valium), and haloperidol (Haldol ) benefit in bringing on a remission of symptoms; the last drug seems to be preferred (Challas & Brauer, 1963; Chapel et al., 1967; Lucas, 1964; Stevens & Blachly, 1966). Initial dosage will vary with age and weight, with increases occurring until symptoms are controlled.

On occasion a child suffering from Sydenham's Chorea or St. Vitus' Dance surfaces in a mental health facility (Halpern, 1974). The peculiarities of behavior can easily mislead the clinician to perceive the problem in purely psychological terms. Early diagnosis and treatment of the rheumatic nature of this disease, including an antibiotic regimen, prevents long-range physical disability, which can occur in up to 75 percent of untreated choreic children. The involuntary choreic movements of the extremities and of the face, not commonly associated with vocal tics, are secondary reactions to streptococcal infection in children from ages five to thirteen years and are more prevalent in girls.

*Case E*

An eight-year-old boy was referred to a community mental health center by his pediatrician after the sudden onset of "nervous" traits and habits. He was said to shake parts of his trunk, blink frequently, jerk his head to one side, and fidget in other unusual ways. Along with this behavior, he had become irritable, was often in tears, and was sleepless. Moreover, he began hiding himself so others could not observe his motions. He had told his parents that he was aware of the movements but that he could not do anything about them. The parents felt that this child had always been a tense youngster.

The history revealed that the boy had had multiple streptococcal throat and ear infections for several years until a tonsillectomy was performed about a year prior to the onset of the current symptoms. Two weeks before the present illness, the patient and a younger brother had complained of earaches but there had been no treatment for this condition.

When the boy was examined the most prominent sign was an involuntary head-shaking tic. There was some minor movement of the shoulders. His overall actions were fast and jerky as if he did not have good control over his body. All laboratory tests were normal except for an elevated AS-O titer which was presumptive evidence for a previous streptococcal infection. A diagnosis of Sydenham's Chorea or St. Vitus' Dance was entertained, and a course of penicillin was prescribed by the pediatrician. About three months after the onset of the symptoms, all involuntary movements had virtually disappeared. The boy's functioning had returned to its premorbid condition of inoffensiveness.

Several British authors have reported successful treatment of stutterers with haloperidol (Haldol) (Barker, 1975; Wells & Malcolm, 1971).

### Phobic States

The treatment of phobic children with antidepressant drugs appears to be practiced more commonly in Great Britain (Kelly et al., 1970) than in the United States, where psychotherapeutic or behavior management methods are preferred. A report about a multidiscipline treatment program of school-phobic children (Gittelman-Klein and Klein, 1971) revealed that imipramine (Tofranil) in dosages of 100-200 mg per day was superior to placebo in obviating the principal symptom. However, the high dosage required introduces risks of side effects, which makes this approach an alternative only after other methods have been unsuccessful. Librium was used successfully to return children to school by one investigator (D'Amato, 1962).

### Learning Problems

There is a growing emphasis on the search for drug-facilitated learning or specific help for the underachieving or learning disabled child. The psychic energizers such as methylphenidate (Ritalin) and pemoline (Cylert) in particular seemed to have some effect on cognitive functioning (Alexandris & Lundell, 1968; Page et al., 1974; Sprague et al., 1970; Rapoport et al., 1974). Even for hypoactive and schizoid children with learning problems, stimulants may be effective in ameliorating some of the dysfunction arising out of subtle developmental deviations (Fish, 1971). Nonetheless, the long-term appropriateness of drug use for this purpose requires further investigation before psychopharmacologic therapy for special learning handicaps can be recommended. Antidepressants have been given to high school underachievers with good results, although it is not certain whether the mood-elevating property or the mild tranquilization or both are responsible (Splitter & Kaufman, 1966). If the claims for improvement in this complex target symptom by any number of chemical agents can be believed, there need hardly be any young person who should not progress on one or another medication. Only the major tranquilizers, like chlorpromazine (Thorazine), have actually been found to have a deleterious influence on learning (Baker, 1968; Hartlage, 1965; McAndrew et al., 1972).

Whenever clinicians use medication as a major intervention strategy, they must pay special attention to the potential for serious side effects. Children in a state of development and generally passive-recipients of whatever adults consider important are doubly at risk. Tables 9–1 through 9–4 list a number of potential side effects that can occur when treating emotional and mental problems with pharmacotherapy. *Physicians' Desk Reference* provides information on probable, possible, and infrequent side effects of all Federal Food and Drug Administration approved medications. The list of side effects found in the PDR can be unnecessarily frightening or overwhelming for the nonmedically oriented clinician.

The Food and Drug Administration routinely surveys registered physicians regarding the side effects of prescribed medication reported by their patients. The list of published side effects is based upon this survey and thus includes a number of infrequently occurring side effects. For example, the 1981 PDR informs the practitioner not to use Ritalin in children below the age of six. However, this drug has been used rather successfully in a number of preschoolers where the risks of not using the drug far outweighed the possible side effects (Halpern, 1977).

The *Physicians' Desk Reference* should not be looked upon as scripture, but as a *reference guide* to assist—not substitute—for clinical judgment.

## TERMINOLOGY

The busy practitioner uses language, especially shorthand versions, as a way of expediting communication. Unfortunately, for those who do not have the "code book," mystification rather than clarification results. The following list presents a number of often-used phrases and how they are commonly abbreviated:

| *Abbreviation* | *Meaning* |
|---|---|
| 1. gr or G. | gram |
| 2. mg or mgm | milligram |
| 3. kg | kilogram |
| 4. stat | immediately |
| 5. p.o. | by mouth |
| 6. i.v. | intravenous injection |
| 7. i.m. | intramuscular injection |
| 8. hs | at bedtime |
| 9. a.c. | before meals |
| 10. p.c. | after meals |
| 11. q.h. | once an hour |

| | |
|---|---|
| 12. q.d. | once a day |
| 13. b.i.d. | twice a day |
| 14. t.i.d. | three times a day |
| 15. q.i.d. | four times a day |
| 16. prn or p.r.n. | as needed |
| 17. amp. | ampule |
| 18. cap. | capsules |
| 19. susp. | suspension |
| 20. tab. | tablets |
| 21. inj. | injection |
| 22. supp. | suppository |

## SUMMARY

The purpose of this very detailed review has been to acquaint the nonmedically oriented practitioner with a number of the important parameters of chemotherapy. Nomenclature, abbreviations, actions, generic and trade names, and side effects were discussed. Some knowledge or experience with psychotropic drugs, however, is no substitute for medical training:

> The assertion that persons with no medical training and relatively little experience can manage drugs effectively is dangerous nonsense. Amateur drug therapists can be disastrous. (Hollister, 1974).

The nonmedically trained practitioner is wise to have at lease one close working relationship with a medically oriented specialist—preferably, but not necessarily, a psychiatrist. Such a person should be available for consultation and evaluation of patients who you believe could benefit from medication as an adjunct to your treatment program.

Some medically oriented referral sources, such as internists and pediatricians, prefer collaborating with their nonmedically trained colleagues regarding the total care of the patient. They feel quite comfortable prescribing psychotropic medications while leaving the psychotherapeutic strategies up to you. Occasional phone contacts regarding any side effects of medication and observations regarding the effectiveness of the medication and progress of the treatment in general are appreciated by the referring physician, cement closer working relationships, and can stimulate new referrals. At times your opinion may be sought regarding the type of drug to prescribe. Physicians who solicit my suggestions are generally receptive. However, when not requested for an opinion concerning what medication to prescribe, silence is the best policy.

# Appendix 9–A

## Chemotherapy References*


Abrahams, D. Treatment of encopresis with imipramine. *American Journal of Psychiatry,* 119, 801–892, 1963.

Alexandris, A. & Lundell, F. Effect of thioridazine, amphetamine and placebo on the hyperkinetic syndrome and cognitive area in mentally deficient children. *The Canadian Medical Association Journal,* 98, 92–96, 1968.

Anders, R.F. & Weinstein, P. Sleep and its disorders in infants and children: A review. *Journal of Pediatrics,* 50, 311–324, 1972.

Annell, A.L. Lithium in the treatment of children and adolescents. *Acta Psychiatrica Scandinavica,* 207, 19–30, 1969. Supplement.

Arnold, L.E., Kirilcuk, V., Corson, S.A., & Corson, E.O'L. Levoamphetamine and dextroamphetamine: Differential effect on aggression and hyperkinesis in children and dogs. *American Journal of Psychiatry,* 130, 165–170, 1973.

Baker, R.R. The effects of psychotropic drugs on psychological testing. *Psychological Bulletin,* 69, 377–387, 1968.

Barker, P. Haloperidol. *Journal of Child Psychology and Psychiatry,* 16, 169–172, 1975.

Beck, L., Langford, W.S., Mackay, M. & Sum, G. Childhood chemotherapy and later drug abuse and growth curve: A follow-up study of 30 adolescents. *American Journal of Psychiatry,* 132, 436–438, 1975.

Bellman, M. Studies on encopresis. *Acta Paediatrica Scandinavica Supplement,* 170, 1–151, 1966.


*These references accompany the material presented earlier in this chapter.

Berg, I. & Jones, K.V. Functional faecal incontinence in children. *Archives of the Diseases of Childhood,* 39, 465–472, 1964.

Bradley, C. The behavior of children receiving benzedrine. *American Journal of Psychiatry,* 94, 577–585, 1937.

Bradley, C. Benzedrine and dexedrine in the treatment of children's behavior disorders. *Pediatrics.* 5, 24–36, 1950.

Brown, D., Winsberg, B.G., Bialer, I. & Press, M. Imipramine therapy and seizures: Three children treated for hyperactive behavior disorders. *American Journal of Psychiatry,* 130, 210–213, 1974.

Call, J.D., Christianson, M., Penrose, F.R. & Backlar, M. Psychogenic megacolon in three preschool boys. A study of etiology through collaborative treatment of child and parents. *American Journal of Orthopsychiatry,* 33, 923–928, 1963.

Campbell, M., Fish, B., Korein, J., Shapiro, T., Collins, P., & Koh, C. Lithium and chlorpromazine: A controlled crossover study of hyperactive severely disturbed young children. *Journal of Autism and Childhood Schizophrenia,* 2, 234–263, 1972a.

Campbell, S.B., Douglas, V.I., & Morgenstern, G. Cognitive styles in hyperactive children and the effect of methylphenidate. *Journal of Child Psychology and Psychiatry,* 12, 55–67, 1971.

Challas, G., & Brauer, W. Tourette's disease: Relief of symptoms with R1625. *American Journal of Psychiatry,* 120, 283–284, 1963.

Chapel, J.L., Brown, N., & Jenkins, R.L. Tourette's disease: Symptomatic relief with haloperidol. *American Journal of Psychiatry,* 121, 608–610, 1967.

Conners, C.K. Psychological effects of stimulant drugs in children with minimal brain dysfunction. *Pediatrics,* 49, 707–708, 1972.

Conners, C.K., Taylor, E., Meo, G., Kurtz, M.A. & Fournier, M. Magnesium pemoline and dextroamphetamine: A controlled study in children with minimal brain dysfunction. *Psychopharmacologia,* 26, 321–336, 1972.

Cytryn, L., McKnew, D.H., Logue, M. & Desai, R.B. Biochemical correlates of affective disorders in children. *Archives of General Psychiatry,* 31, 659–661, 1974.

Dally, P. & Sargant, W. Treatment and outcome of anorexia nervosa. *British Medical Journal,* 2, 793–795, 1966.

D'Amata, G. Chlordiazepoxide in management of school phobia. *Diseases of the Nervous System,* 23, 292–295, 1962.

Eisenberg, L. Principles of drug therapy in child psychiatry with special reference to stimulant drugs. *American Journal of Orthopsychiatry,* 41, 371–379, 1971.

Eisenberg, L. The hyperkinetic child and stimulant drugs. *New England Journal of Medicine,* 287, 249–250, 1972.

Eisenberg, L., Lachman, R., Molling, P.A., Lockner, A., Mizelle, J.D. & Conners, C.K. A psychopharmacologic experiment in a training school for delinquent boys: Methods, problems, findings. *American Journal of Orthopsychiatry,* 33, 431, 447, 1963.

Feinstein, S.C. & Wolpert, E.A. Juvenile manic-depressive illness. Clinical and therapeutic considerations. *Journal of the American Academy of Child Psychiatry,* 12, 123--136, 1973.

Fish, B. The "one child, one drug" myth of stimulants in hyperkinesis: Importance of diagnostic categories in evaluating treatment. *Archives of General Psychiatry,* 25, 193–203, 1971.

Freeman, R.D. Drug effects on learning in children. A selective review of the past thirty years. *Journal of Special Education,* 1, 17–44, 1966.

Frommer, E.A. Treatment of childhood depression with antidepressant drugs. *British Medical Journal,* 1, 729–732, 1967.

Galdston, R. Mind over matter: Observations on 50 patients hospitalized with anorexia nervosa. *Journal of the American Academy of Child Psychiatry,* 13, 246–263, 1974.

Gavanski, M. Treatment of non-retentive secondary encopresis with imipramine and psychotherapy. *Canadian Medical Association Journal,* 104, 46–48, 1971.

Ginn, S., & Hohman, L. The use of dextroamphetamine in severe behavior problems of children. *Southern Medical Journal,* 46, 1124–1127, 1953.

Gittelman-Klein, R., & Klein, D. Controlled imipramine treatment of school phobia. *Archives of General Psychiatry,* 25, 204–207, 1971.

Grinspoon, L., & Singer, S.B. Amphetamines in the treatment of hyperkinetic children, *Harvard Educational Review,* 43, 515–555, 1973.

Halpern, W.I. St. Vitus' Dance: Psychological symptoms as masquerade for physical illness in children. *Bulletin of the Rochester Mental Health Center,* 6, 2–10, 1974.

Hartlage, L.C. Effects of chlorpromazine on learning. *Psychological Bulletin,* 64, 235–245, 1965.

Kelly, D., Guirguis, W., Frommer, E., Mitchell-Heggs, N. & Sargant, W. Treatment of phobic states with antidepressants. A retrospective study of 246 patients. *British Journal of Psychiatry,* 116, 387–398, 1970.

Koupernik, C. Chemotherapy in child psychiatry. *British Medical Journal,* 3, 345–346, 1972.

Laufer, M.W. Long-term management and some follow-up findings on the use of drugs with minimal cerebral syndromes. *Journal of Learning Disabilities,* 4, 54–58, 1971a.

Laufer, M.W. Long-term management and some follow-up findings on the use of drugs with minimal brain syndromes. *Journal of Learning Disabilities,* 4, 518–522, 1971b.

Lorber, J. Obesity in childhood: A controlled trial of anorectic drugs. *Archives of Diseases in Childhood,* 41, 309–312, 1966.

Lucas, A.R. Gilles de la Tourette's disease in children: Treatment with phenothiazine drugs, *American Journal of Psychiatry,* 121, 606–608, 1964.

McAndrew, J.B., Case, Q. & Treffert, D.A. Effects of prolonged phenothiazine intake on psychotic and other hospitalized children. *Journal of Autism and Childhood Schizophrenia,* 2, 75–91, 1972.

Margolis, L.H. Control of enuresis with imipramine. *American Journal of Psychiatry,* 119, 269–270, 1962.

Martin, G.I., & Zang, P. Electrocardiographic monitoring of enuretic children receiving therapeutic doses of imipramine. *American Journal of Psychiatry,* 132, 540–542, 1975.

Mattson, R.H., & Calverley, J.R. Dextroamphetamine-sulfate-induced dyskinesias. *Journal of the American Medical Association,* 204, 108–110, 1968.

Millichap, J.G. Drugs in management of hyperkinetic and perceptually-handicapped children. *Journal of the American Medical Association,* 206, 1527–1530, 1968.

Muellner, S.R. Development of urinary control in children: A new concept in cause, prevention and treatment of primary enuresis. *Journal of Urology,* 84, 714–716, 1960.

Munster, A.J., Stanley, A.M., & Saunders, J.C. Imipramine (Tofranil) in the treatment of enuresis. *American Journal of Psychiatry,* 118, 76–77, 1961.

Page, J.G., Janicki, R.S., Bernstein, J.E., Curran, C.F. & Michelli, F.A. Pemoline (Cylert) in the treatment of childhood hyperkinesis. *Journal of Learning Disabilities,* 7, 498–503, 1974.

Poussaint, A.F. & Ditman, K.S. A controlled study of imipramine (Tofranil) in the treatment of childhood enuresis. *Journal of Pediatrics,* 67, 283–290, 1965.

Quinn, P.O. & Rapoport, J. One-year follow-up of hyperactive boys treated with imipramine or methylphenidate. *American Journal of Psychiatry,* 132, 241–245, 1975.

Rapoport, J., Quinn, P.O., Bradbard, G., Riddle, K.D. & Brooks, E. Imipramine and methylphenidate treatments of hyperactive boys. A double-blind comparison. *Archives of General Psychiatry,* 30, 789–793, 1974.

Safer, D.J. & Allen, R.P. Factors influencing the suppressant effects of two stimulant drugs on the growth of hyperactive children. *Pediatrics,* 51, 660–667, 1973.

Safer, D., Allen, R. & Barr, E. Depression of growth in hyperactive children on stimulant drugs. *New England Journal of Medicine,* 287, 217–220, 1972.

Schleifer, M., Weiss, G., Cohen, N., Elman, M., Cvejic, J. & Kruger, E. Hyperactivity in preschoolers and the effect of methylphenidate. *American Journal of Orthopsychiatry,* 45, 38–50, 1975.

Schnackenberg, R.C. Caffeine as a substitute for Schedule II stimulants in hyperkinetic children. *American Journal of Psychiatry,* 130, 796–798, 1973.

Splitter, S.R. & Kaufman, M.A. A new treatment for underachieving adolescents: Psychotherapy combined with nortriptyline medication. *Psychosomatics,* 7, 171–174, 1966.

Sprague, R., Barnes, K. & Werry, J. Methylphenidate and thioridazine: Learning, activity, and behavior in emotionally disturbed boys. *American Journal of Orthopsychiatry,* 40, 615–628, 1970.

Stevens, J.R. & Blachly, P.H. Successful treatment of the maladies des tics. Gilles de la Tourette's syndrome. *American Journal of Diseases of Children,* 112, 541–545, 1966.

Tec, L. Unexpected effects in children treated with imipramine. *American Journal of Psychiatry,* 120, 603, 1963.

Tolstrup, K. The treatment of anorexia nervosa in childhood and adolescence. *Journal of Child Psychology and Psychiatry,* 16, 75–78, 1975.

Weiss, G., Minde, K., Douglas, V., Werry, J., & Sykes, D. Comparison of the effects of chlorpromazine, dextroamphetamine, and methylphenidate on the behavior and intellectual function of hyperactive children. *Canadian Medical Association Journal,* 104, 20–25, 1971a.

Weiss, G., Minde, K. & Werry, J.S. Studies on the hyperactive child VIII. Five-year follow-up. *Archives of General Psychiatry,* 24, 409–414, 1971b.

Wells, G.H. & Malcolm, M.T. Controlled trial of the treatment of 36 stutterers. *British Journal of Psychiatry,* 119, 603–604, 1971.

Yoss, R.E. & Daly, D.D. Narcolepsy in children. *Pediatrics,* 25, 1025–1033, 1960.

Chapter 10

# Intervention Strategies

# 10

Prior to the nineteenth century, mental health intervention tactics were rooted in religious and mystical practices. Deviant or "strange" behavior was looked upon as the work of the devil—banishment, sequestering, or death were the treatment tactics of choice.

Advances in the biological sciences during the nineteenth century led to changing views of mental illness and its cures. Freud's work emphasized the importance of unconscious mental processes in understanding irrational actions, disturbed thoughts, and symptoms of emotional illness. Once one grasped the psychodynamics and manipulations of symbolic communication of the disturbed, it was thought that interpretation or clarification of the connection between act, thought, and distorted perceptions would relieve anxiety and symptom. Today, dynamic intervention has become an important intervention strategy helpful to mental health practitioners whether or not they practice psychoanalysis.

However, unfulfilled promises (Eysenck, 1965; Levitt, 1971; Leventhal and Weinberger, 1975; Kissel, 1974), the changing sociopolitical milieu that favored an autocratic-oriented technocratic leadership (Halpern and Kissel, 1976), and advances in medical management of emotional illness (Hollister, 1974) led clinicians to search for intervention strategies not rooted in a psychodynamic formulation of the mind. Practical, efficient, and behaviorally oriented intervention strategies emerged as an answer to the dissatisfaction of clinicians with the dynamic model.

Currently, the journeyman practitioner has an abundance of therapeutic strategies and techniques available. In this chapter we will examine two major strategies in detail—the psychodynamic and the behavior-cognitive—which provide techniques, principles, and direction to the clinician. The medical (chemotherapy) elements of treatment have been explored in Chapter 9.

## PSYCHODYNAMIC STRATEGIES

Since psychodynamic psychotherapy looks to psychoanalytic thinking about the nature of the human psyche, a brief description of Freudian and neo-Freudian postulates is in order. Halpern and Kissel (1976) have summarized the position as follows:

> **The Freudian Approach**
>
> The genetic point of view of human development is the rockbed of psychoanalytic theory. It formulates a biologic timetable of libidinal and organizational development in circumscribed and sequential psychosocial stages, provided the necessary environmental conditions exist at the proper time for the unfolding of optimal growth potentials. Problems arise when there are deficiencies in drive or in stimulus tolerance, or the infant and child are subjected to improper care—whether in the form of understimulation, overstimulation, disorganization, trauma-fixating development, or even bringing on regression to earlier stages. The negotiation of later stages is contingent on the successful passage through the preceding ones. Failure to do so produces personality flaws related to that period of developmental life in which the anlage for further emotional maturation was aborted. Therapeutic intervention must then deal with the possibility of bringing that individual through an experience that resembles the stepping stone sequences of his psychological upbringing.
>
> At no point in extrauterine life is the human organism free of the contrary tensions associated with self-gratification and socialization. The baby already must learn to deal with two masters, a process that eventually will govern him from within. On the one hand is the powerful drive for preservation of the self, that is, of the instinctual drives of hunger and libidinal sexuality, while on the other is the social code that prescribes how these drives will be controlled and expressed. The dynamic point of view holds that the intrapsychic conflict arising out of this distinctly human condition is a basic attribute of psychic activity. It assumes that although conflict-free child rearing is unavoidable and even disastrous if it were possible, the quantity and quality of the conflict experiences are primary in giving impetus to a potentially healthy or abnormal reaction to the tension.
>
> In order to understand the individual's regulating or feedback mechanism in the intrapsychic conflict model, another postulate

had to be added. Thus the economic point of view in psychoanalytic theory speaks of psychological energy which is expended in a free flowing manner until checked by experience and redirected or "bound" by the influence of sensory and psychic pain. The pleasure principle espouses a primary process of free flowing energy seeking discharge, whereas the reality principle holds that the energy is reflected back on the organismic system as a secondary process. This occurs when the primal discharge of energy in and of itself becomes less rewarding than a modified version that requires the partial use of the energy for restraint or other secondary behavior. Learning, therefore, can proceed only if there is exposure to the reality principle, that is, to situations that are sufficiently denying and frustrating to the young organism to force him to find alternate routes for gratification.

The topographic point of view acknowledges that experience is both amorphous and particular. It explains the primitive and sophisticated as something that is unified in the makeup of each person by postulating unconscious, preconscious, and conscious subsystems of the psyche. Each person is a store of life forces and of the experiential processes that accrue through time and space. The leading edge to this reservoir of energy is the conscious, a state of self-awareness that permits the individual to perform at a level that he can rationalize. Most of his inner experience remains hidden from understanding or even awareness under normal conditions, except in dreams or reverie. However, the unconscious, as this state of undifferentiated inner experience is called, intrudes constantly on the conscious decision-making process in ways that—with some effort—can be analyzed. Through the medium of the preconscious, a sort of screening or mediating state, the individual has access to influences from the unconscious that may have some pertinence to an understanding of the self.

The structural point of view, yet another tenet of psychoanalysis, tries to answer the question of how the individual secures an internal balance of forces. The life forces of hunger and libido are designated as id or primitive drives that assert themselves heedlessly, presumably for the sake of survival. However, experience soon teaches that personal survival is also predicated on the child's ability to please adults. This he accomplishes by learning the values, prohibitions and ideals of his parents and of their society. Eventually he makes these judgments his own in the formation of a superego, a potent check on the expression of instinctual forces. To both moderate between these two opposing interests and to make the necessary executive decisions, in favor of action or inhibition, stands the ego, which is all those functions at the command of the individual that subserve his information processing and reasoning capacity. Not all ego functions are devoted to arbitration between id and superego. Many are conflict-free or autonomous sensorimotor, behavioral, and integrative processes for gaining mastery over the environment. Methods for dealing with human problems have to distinguish between those stemming primarily from miscarriages in meshing impulse life with conscience and those emanating from deficiencies in autonomous coping functions. White (1963) postulates that the child's play exploration is inherently satisfying in the here and now and that it need not be secondary to drive reduction, to learning, or to conflict resolution. Yet, play is also sensitive to poorly resolving problems so that it can become a vehicle for the expression of disturbance.

In addition to the distinctions made between unconscious and conscious within the individual, an interface has to be recognized between inner and outer reality. The adaptive point of view in psychoanalytic thinking posits a continuous process whereby the individual internalizes external reality in order to achieve a workable relationship to it. The more clearly a person distinguishes his experiential roots in himself and in the world outside of himself, the better is his position to develop a creative accommodation to his existential condition. All therapy must at least perform a service of fostering sufficient reality testing to keep the individual in touch with what comes from self and what from nonself if it hopes to fulfill its promise of being a healing influence.

Finally, the psychosocial or epigenetic point of view sees an interdigitation between the developing child and the social institutions that in itself forms a unity through which mutual regulation evolves. In other words, growth occurs not only within the organism but also in a psychosocial context. The fit between the two contributes to the pace and style of both individual development and to societal evolving. Therefore individual treatment must always keep in mind the presence of the social and cultural matrix of forces in personal problems.

A therapy based on a multifaceted understanding of personality development and adaptation must, by necessity, either delve deeply into the psychological makeup of the person in order to bring about a realignment of contending psychic forces or select a specific deficit for strengthening so that a better chance for personal problem solving can come about. As a result there have been clinicians who focused on the global effects of therapy and those who concentrated on modifying selective parts of the personality or just achieving symptom relief.

**The Doctor-Patient Relationship**

Whether the focus of the therapy is on repressed impulses—sexual or hostile; social attitudes such as moving toward, away from, or against others; a search for influencing archetype; an examination of overcompensations and strivings for superiority; or a coming to grips with basic anxiety resulting from the birth trauma, all dynamic therapies place a premium on the relationship established between doctor and patient, and a dynamic-diagnostic appraisal of the patient resulting in a plan of treatment. In each case, the therapist must decide whether to provide a supportive or uncovering type of relationship.

*The Supportive Role*

In the supportive role the therapist provides a benign and permissive environment. In such a relationship some regressive needs to be dependent can thus be satisfied and thereby reduce the need for such gratification through symptoms; a free discussion of practical problems stimulates patients to use their intellectual capacities; catharsis helps to reduce tension and anxiety levels leading patients to feel better about themselves (Patterson, 1980). The status of the therapist and the relationship provided help to instill confidence in the patient. Attentive listening is a major technique used by dynamic therapists when engaging in supportive therapy.

Psychotherapists engage in attentive listening by attending to the verbal and nonverbal communication and commenting upon some refractory tendency, pointing out a discrepancy between intention (wishes and attitudes) and execution (behavior), or reflecting on their own puzzlement regarding a patient's comments or actions.

The focus is on incongruities between what is said and how a comment is stated. After listening to a mother describe a number of major battles between her teen-age daughter and herself, the therapist says to the woman: "You keep insisting Sally take more responsibility, yet when she suggests her own way of doing something, you seem to find fault."

This is another example of attentive listening during a family therapy session:

*Mother:* Occasionally I get mad.

*Children:* You're always mad.

*Father (bored voice):* I would agree Jane gets mad on occasion.

*Children:* Aw, come on, Dad!

*Therapist (to father):* What happens when you get mad?

*Father:* I try not to get angry.

*Mother (to father):* You can say that again! (*to therapist*): He never says anything to the children when they do wrong so I get mad for both of us, yell at the kids, and then have to run to the bathroom because I get these excruciating stomach pains. I'm so upset I usually have to lie down after that."

*Father: (sighs and looks at floor while his wife sobs).*

*Therapist (to father):* "Yes?"

*Father:* "Nothing."

*Father (to children):* "I say what I think, don't I?"

*Children: (mumble, look at floor):* "Sometimes."

*Therapist:* "What do you think would happen if you got upset and expressed anger?"

*Father:* "I don't know. I guess my wife would get upset, cry, or have one of her stomachaches and have to lie down."

*Therapist:* "It sounds like you're afraid to show your feelings, especially when you get mad."

In his last comment, the therapist reflects on the incongruity between the father's attitude during the discussion and his behavior.

A related supportive technique is reflexive explorations. This is very succinctly described by Choca (1980) in the following way:

> Reflexive explorations are statements in which the therapist rephrases what the client said. When done well, the rephrasing a) adds some meaning to what the client said and b) encourages the client to go on exploring his or her feelings.

An example may be the following interaction:

C: I had a very hard time when my wife left me.

T: Yes, I can see by your expression that you still have a lot of feelings about it.

Notice the therapist is adding his or her perception of the client's present state and leaving the comment open-ended in a way that encourages the client to continue.

This is an extremely useful technique that can be used frequently. Choca feels, however, that it can also be overused: its goal is to explore and make clients aware of their feelings. The reader should keep this in mind and not use the technique when this goal is not being pursued.

*The Uncovering Role*

Uncovering psychotherapy utilizes techniques such as environmental manipulation, abreaction, defense strengthening, but in addition uses interpretation, insight, and working through.

*Interpretation* is the process whereby the therapist helps the patient relate something occurring in the present with past or seemingly nonrelated events:

Client: I'm tired of not having friends. Each time I think I might be able to get to know somebody and make a friend, something seems to go wrong.

Therapist: Perhaps you have something to do with these breakups.

If an interpretation is to be successful, the patient has to be aware of the present feelings and thoughts in question and the past experience that is being related.

*Insight* is the patient's true (as distinct from merely verbal) understanding of the origins and unconscious dynamics of his or her behavior.

*Working through* is a reexploration of a problem situation, tracing its symbolic meaning to "deep" unconscious sources in order to find a satisfactory solution or adaptation to the problem.

Consider the following case:

The I's, a childless couple, entered therapy during the sixth year of their marriage, presenting themselves as troubled over their inability to have children. The husband was ten years his wife's senior, and they met while working in the same office. She was a secretary in the firm that employed her husband as an office manager. They had married two years after she graduated from high school. Both agreed their sex life together was good, although Mrs. I felt they did not have sex relations frequently enough, while Mr. I suggested that he was not "an animal." It appeared that the husband was a more domineering and assertive person who either minimized or dismissed his wife's suggestions about their marriage or his actions. He also drank more than she liked, although not to excess, and he had a quick temper. Furthermore, he was extremely critical of her housekeeping abilities and seemed to demand more than she felt was reasonable.

While Mrs. I did not openly admit to feeling inferior to her husband, she was constantly asking for his opinion, felt uncomfortable making decisions by herself, and readily called him at work. She leaned on him a great deal and, thus, conformed to the role of a "pretty but helpless wife."

Mrs. I complained that in the last two years she had changed from a bubbling, happy-go-lucky woman to a tense, "shrieking neurotic," who often would tear up during the day and whose hands began trembling at times for no apparent reason. She no longer felt good or confident about herself. Mr. I, on the other hand, seemed to have become somewhat more rigid and compulsive in his activities but was quite content with his marriage. For example, if the paper was not waiting for him when he returned from work, or if he was interrupted before his morning shower, he would erupt in a tirade.

In one of their heated discussions during a therapy session, the therapist turned to Mrs. I and asked where she felt her husband learned to treat her the way he does. Of course, she suggested that it was in the home and the experiences he had with his parents. The rest of the session was spent in a discussion of the husband's early childhood experiences with his parents and the perceptions he had of how his father treated his mother.

Messer and Winokur (1980) have recently presented a case that very clearly illustrates the approach of the dynamically oriented psychotherapist and which will later be used to contrast with behaviorally oriented strategies of intervention.

> Mrs. J, a 37-year-old-mother of two children, is currently separated from her husband and dating another man. For about two years she has had considerable fluctuation of moods and concerns about her adequacy. She alternates between feeling good about herself and feeling very low, depressed, self-blaming, and physically unattractive. During these low periods, she has a strong compulsion to eat and recently gained 20 pounds. The most significant events in her recent history are that her father, to whom she was close, died about ten months ago. She describes her mother as having frustrated her a great deal, as not being well attuned to her

> needs, and as having shifted a lot of the mothering chore to the client's older sister. Her father is described as basically loving, caring, and generous. "I loved him dearly and he loved me." (p. 819)

Messer and Winokur suggest that the dynamically oriented therapist would understand Mrs. J's behavior from an introspective point of view and emphasize private unconscious events such as repressed hostility toward the father, explore the symbolic meaning of overeating, and focus on the client's feelings of phoniness and its meaning in the context of her life history.

## COGNITIVE-BEHAVIOR STRATEGIES

Cognitive-behavior modification approaches to healing consist of an understanding of human suffering that differs from the dynamic approach we have just considered. They embody a large assortment of techniques and principles.

In a relatively brief period of time, voluminous literature has emerged on behavior and cognitive approaches to the treatment of mental and emotional illness. Comprehensive reviews of the appropriateness, effectiveness, and application of behavior modification can be found in the writings of Bergin and Suinn (1975), Graziano (1971, 1978), Krasner (1971), O'Leary and Wilson (1975), and Yates (1970).

Although behavior therapy and cognitive therapy have somewhat different theoretical notions, in practice behaviorally oriented therapists borrow freely from their more cognitively oriented brethren.

We will consider each approach as if the two are purely different strategies although in fact there are a variety of behavior and cognitive therapies.

### Behavior Therapy

Despite divergent theories or techniques, all behavior-oriented therapists subscribe to a common code that can be encompassed by the following three key concepts:

- Overt behavior rather than underlying covert conditions is the major focus of therapy.
- Knowledge of the principles of learning theory with particular emphasis on the systematic application of reinforcement and extinction is central to conceptualizing human behavior.
- Behavior that is to be modified has to be observable and specific so that it can be counted and documented.

It follows that the therapist working with a patient within this framework will focus on the stimulating characteristics of the external environment and attempt to systematically manipulate those stimulating conditions that are believed to be maladaptive.

Referring back to the case of Mrs. J (Messer and Winokur, 1980), a behavioral approach would consist of the following:

> The client might be asked to self-monitor the antecedents of her eating behavior but noting the conditions preceding her overeating (e.g., after an argument with her boyfriend, when bored, etc.) and her associated thoughts ("It's only a sandwich," "I deserve a reward," "I feel unhappy") and asked to keep track of the target behavior by counting caloric intake and weight gain or loss. With this information in hand, the therapist might then suggest a plan to decrease caloric intake and to increase amount of exercise. He or she would also point to the client's rationalization for overeating and encourage her to stop deluding herself as to the eventual consequences, namely, weight gain. The rationale for this intervention would be to improve the client's self-esteem and sense of control over one area of her life. (p. 80)

Another example shows how this orientation is applicable to marriage counseling:

Mrs. G complained that the evening meal was a disaster. She and her husband agreed that from the moment he walked into the house until the children went to bed their family was in a state of turmoil. Mr. G complained that upon returning from work he felt assaulted by his seven- and ten-year-old daughters. As a result of this, he and his wife often argued and then went to bed angry. Mrs. G was rather unsympathetic to his comments and reminded him that he should be more understanding of her feelings because she gets that type of behavior all day long. Furthermore, she added that when her husband comes home she would like some attention from him because she often feels starved for adult stimulation. Mr. G characterized himself as an intense person who finds his work both exhilarating and taxing. Thus he felt the necessity for time to unwind when he gets home before entering "the family circus." His wife thought it was unfortunate that they were unable to afford "help."

The therapist suggested the couple keep a week's record of the number of incidents of the type they had been discussing. In addition, they were instructed to record precisely the activities that seemed to precipitate such events. At the next meeting, one week later, parents reported four nights of disruptions, i.e., fighting between the child and one parent or arguments between each parent prior to dinner. One night the father was not home, and as usual, on weekends the problem did not exist.

The suggestion was made that both parents relax together for 30 minutes immediately after father comes home from work, talking with one another in the living room and having a cocktail. The girls were to be informed that they could not have mother's or father's attention during that period of time. Dinner was to follow, and the girls were told their father would talk with them about whatever they wished to discuss while dinner was being prepared by the mother.

In addition to viewing a person as a product of learning and conceptualizing neurotic behavior as the neurotic condition, behavior therapists bring a wide variety of specific techniques into the consultation room.

### *Systematic Desensitization*

Systematic desensitization was originally devised for patients who were phobic, but has since been applied to a number of different maladaptive problems associated with intensive anxiety. Classical Pavlovian conditioning provides the theoretical basis for the procedure. Three major operations are involved:

1. The patient is trained in deep relaxation.
2. A habit or anxiety hierarchy is elicited whereby the patient lists in descending order those situations that generate increasing increments of anxiety.
3. The patient is asked to imagine the least disturbing scenes in the hierarchy while relaxed so that they no longer elicit anxiety. He or she then gradually works through the entire list in this fashion.

A 35-year-old male with chronic stress at work was referred by his internist. A preliminary examination revealed the patient found it extremely difficult to relax around persons in authority and was having progressively more difficulty relating to his supervisors at work. Together we constructed an anxiety hierarchy, listing a number of situations that the patient agreed were anxiety producing.

1. Walking past and greeting one of the bosses at work who is only a little older than myself.
2. Walking past and greeting one of the bosses at work who is considerably older than myself—one with gray hair and a gruff but somewhat fatherly demeanor.

3. Encountering one of the bosses who is only a little older than myself in the coffee-break room, where we will have to talk and have coffee together.
4. Encountering one of the bosses who is considerably older than myself—with gray hair and a gruff but somewhat fatherly demeanor—in the coffee-break room, where we will have to talk and have coffee together.
5. Having one of the bosses who is only a little older than myself watch me, without seeming pleased or displeased, while I work.
6. Having one of the bosses who is considerably older than myself—with gray hair and a gruff but somewhat fatherly demeanor—watch me while I work—without seeming pleased or displeased.
7. Having one of the bosses who is only a little older than myself watch me while I work and seeming to be displeased with what I am doing.
8. Having one of the bosses who is considerably older than myself—with gray hair and a gruff but somewhat fatherly demeanor—watch me while I work and seem to be displeased with what I am doing.
9. Having one of the bosses who is only a little older than myself watch me while I work and make a slightly critical comment to me after watching for a while.
10. Having one of the bosses who is considerably older than myself—with gray hair and a gruff but somewhat fatherly demeanor—watch me while I work and make a slightly critical comment to me after watching for a while.
11. Having one of the bosses who is only a little older than myself watch me while I work and make a very critical comment after watching for a while.
12. Having one of the bosses who is considerably older than myself—with gray hair and a gruff but somewhat fatherly demeanor—watch me while I work and make a very critical comment after watching for a while.
13. Attending a conference in the office of one of the bosses who is only a little older than myself to discuss something about my work that should be improved.
14. Attending a conference in the office of one of the bosses who is considerably older than myself—with gray hair and a gruff but somewhat fatherly demeanor—to discuss something about my work that should be improved.
15. Attending a conference with several bosses both young and old to discuss something about my work that should be improved.

Two sessions were spent in teaching the patient deep relaxation using the Jacobson Technique of muscle relaxation, and having him imagine a number of neutral scenes. It took us eight weeks to get through pairing fifteen scenes on the hierarchy with a state of deep relaxation. At a follow-up two months following termination, the patient reported he was having considerably less stress talking with the supervisor but did still find it mildly anxiety producing when presenting to a number of bosses at a conference.

### *Contingency Management*

Operant or instrumental conditioning provides the theoretical basis for a varied number of techniques in which behavior is understood to be controlled by antecedent and consequent events. In a contingency management program, the therapist focuses on the consequences of the patient's actions, that is, the rewards and punishments that follow a certain behavior or are contingent on that behavior.

Contingency management techniques have been used to strengthen existing adaptive behaviors, develop new adaptive behaviors, and eliminate existing inappropriate or maladaptive behaviors.

Mental health practitioners are usually called upon to help a patient overcome the debilitating effects of maladaptive behavior. Satiation, ignoring, learning alternative behavior, and aversion are four techniques that have been found helpful in eliminating inappropriate or maladaptive behaviors.

*Satiation* involves the practice of suggesting and often insisting that a patient continue performing the undesired act until he or she tires of it. For example, insisting a fire-setting child be made to light many matches in quick succession or having a patient with a tic practice the tic for a prolonged period of time.

I have used a variation of this procedure most successfully in families where a young child repeatedly disturbs the parents during the night and ultimately winds up sleeping in the room against their wishes.

I have instructed the parents to inform their children they can wake the parents as often as necessary if they are upset during the evening. The parents are further instructed to comfort the child and then escort him or her back to the room. Usually within a week the child stops disturbing the parents.

Of course, when the behavior in question will result in others being hurt, the satiation technique is not appropriate.

When conditions are arranged so that positive rewards (attention, anger) do not follow the undesirable act, then *extinction* is being used. Matter-of-factly sending children to their room away from family, friends, books, food, and TV is one example of how parents have intuitively made use of this technique.

A hypertensive, middle-aged woman was referred by her internist because she found it exceedingly difficult to tolerate the uncooperativeness of her six- and eight-year-old children. Separate evaluations of the children revealed both of them to be pleasant, bright, and articulate. Evidently they related without difficulty. They each had a number of friends of their own and did well in school.

The mother was particularly troubled by the children's behavior when they returned from school each day as "they entered the house fighting," and she felt this set the tone for the rest of the day until her husband came home for dinner, when things settled down. It was decided to attempt to modify the children's behavior with positive reinforcement for acceptable behavior and extinguishing unacceptable acts through ignoring such behavior.

The mother was instructed to sit down with both children and discuss with them her concerns regarding their behavior of yelling at each other, shouting, and crying as they entered the house from school. In addition, she was asked to enlist their involvement in the program by determining with them what special things they would like. The eight-year-old expressed an interest in models and matchbox cars while the six-year-old wanted costume jewelry and play makeup.

The mother informed the children they would both be given a check for each school day they entered the house without fighting with each other. If either one yelled, screamed, or cried, neither would receive a check.

Three weeks later the mother was glowing in her reports of success, but wondered if she would have to give the children "toys for the rest of their lives." She was then instructed to require more work from the children for the same reward, that is 8 checks, and after two additional successful weeks, 10 checks for the car or jewelry. In addition to praising her for the progress she had made with the program, the therapist stressed that it was important for her not only to continually praise the children for their efforts but also to help them see the functional benefits from cooperating with each other, such as playing with each other when friends were not available, more readily sharing toys, and having more fun together.

By far the best way to try to help a patient eliminate some maladaptive action is to suggest *alternative behaviors*. The aim is to help the patient find some behavior that is incompatible with the maladaptive behavior, reward it, and thus, while it is being performed, the maladaptive act cannot take place.

With the technique of *aversion* the patient is required to act in a more adaptive, that is, prosocial way in order to terminate an aversive situation. This approach has been used to treat patients whose behavior disorders are highly self-reinforcing, i.e., sexual disorders, alcoholism, and some forms of self-mutilation.

*Assertiveness Training*

Many clients have serious difficulty asserting themselves in social situations or at work. Their inability may be the result of inhibiting strong anxiety or it may be caused by a lack of social skill.

Graziano (1978) has characterized assertiveness training as consisting of "(1) a specification of the conditions under which problematic non-assertive behavior occurs and (2) systematic training to teach specified, alternative behavior, in this instance assertive behavior" (p. 34). *Behavioral rehearsal,* which is a role-playing technique, is often used in assertiveness training. The client can rehearse playing a role, i.e., making assertive statements, while the therapist reacts appropriately. After successful coaching in being more assertive in the role playing, the client is encouraged to apply the newly learned assertiveness in real-life situations.

*Contingency Contracting*

The technique of contingency contracting is also based on the learning principle that behavior is strengthened or weakened depending on the consequences. While appropriate for all stages of development, contingency contracting is particularly relevant for the handling of conflicts between adolescents and their parents:

- It places the relationship at the heart of the problem.
- It provides recognition of the growing maturity of the youth.
- It upholds the parents' rights to expect something of the child.
- It helps to open up communication among all parties by defusing a highly charged situation.

When working out a behavioral contract with a family, the consequences need to have a positive valence for the participants. The therapist sits down with the "combatants" and writes out a "legal" contract to be signed by all parties. The contract will state specifically who is to do what, the consequences of the action, and the period of time (or job) for which the contract is in force. Exhibit 10–1 presents a sample behavior contract.

A mother requested an evaluation of her teen-age daughter, who had been in and out of individual psychotherapy for a considerable number of years because she was doing poorly in school. A number of deficiency reports had been sent home, suggesting that while the girl was well above average in intelligence, she was failing almost all of her tenth grade subjects. During an initial family interview, it became clear that it was extremely difficult for family members to communicate with one another. They tended to interrupt each other and listened with preconceived ideas. The daughter accused her parents of constantly nagging while they defended their behavior because of her deficiency reports.

**Exhibit 10–1** Sample Behavior Contract

BEHAVIOR CONTRACT

(I/We), ______________________________ hereby declare that
(I/We) will ______________________________
(does what)
This job will be considered successful ______________________________
(how well)
______________________________
(signed)

For the successful completion of the above job you may
______________________________
(reward)
Date Signed:
Date Completed: ______________ ______________________________
(signed)

Behavioral contracting was suggested to alleviate the problem. As a first step the therapist stated that a contract be worked out around the parents' nagging and the girl's homework behavior. Each family member was asked to give some thought to the matter separately. At the next meeting they wrote a contract that stated that the girl would do one hour of homework each day and that the homework would be considered successful when the number of problems she agreed to do matched the assignment she brought home and had shown to her parents prior to beginning her homework. The parents agreed furthermore that they would not remind her of her work, but did agree to permit her to stay out an additional two hours on Friday nights for the successful completion of four homework assignments. That is, if she did her work from Monday through Thursday, then on that Friday or possibly Saturday evening, she could stay out the additional two hours. All parties signed the contract and the therapist signed as a witness.

The following week, parents commented that the house was considerably quieter, and their daughter told the therapist with a smile that she chose to see the "late movie with friends" rather than going to the early show.

### *Thought Stopping*

Thought stopping, a procedure introduced by Cautela and Wisocki (1977), can be very successfully applied when treating patients who are obsessed with thoughts that are unrealistic, unproductive, and anxiety or depression arousing. Cautela and Wisocki (1977) have provided a very exacting description of the procedure.

The therapist asks the client to list any disturbing thoughts which he/she feels are out of his/her control. Special emphasis is placed on any overt and covert behaviors which could have harmful social consequences, such as robbery, murder, rape, etc. Each item on the list is translated into a concrete statement in the client's own vocabulary.

Once the target thoughts are agreed upon, the therapist and client discuss the rationale for eliminating them. This discussion usually centers around the notion that such self-statements are detrimental to constructive action and often lead to maladaptive overt behaviors, such as withdrawal from social events, etc. (If the client complains particularly of maladaptive approach behaviors, such as overeating, smoking, excessive alcohol intake, the therapist inquires about anticipatory thoughts antecedent to the behavior, e.g., saying to oneself, "I'd love to have a drink," and explains that the elimination of such thoughts should reduce the frequency of the target behavior.) Finally, the therapist discusses the self-control aspects of the TS procedure, indicating to the client that once he/she has learned TS, it will remain useful at any future time.

The verbatim instructions given to a client as a demonstration of the TS technique are as follows:

> Now sit back, relax, and close your eyes. In a few seconds, I'm going to say the word "go." As soon as I say the word "go," I want you to deliberately think this thought: (example: "The future is hopeless"). As soon as you begin the thought with the words, "The future," signal me by raising your right index finger. Do you understand the instructions? Okay. Lean back. Relax. Are you ready? Go.

As soon as the client raises a finger, the therapist loudly shouts "stop," usually producing a startle response. The client will then open his or her eyes and the therapist asks about the experience. The client may respond in a number of ways. Some typical responses are: "Well, you startled me"; "I got scared"; "You interrupted the thought." If the client doesn't mention that the thought itself disappeared, the therapist prompts for that specific response and then goes on to explain that a person cannot think of two things at the same time. A second trial is given during which the therapist does not shout "stop" immediately upon the client's signal but waits about one sec. before evoking the startle response. Again, inquiry is made about the experience and the client usually responds that the thought disappeared.

In explaining the need for the client to learn the technique for his or her own use, the therapist gives the following instructions: "I'm going to ask you to close your eyes again, but this time I'm not going to yell stop. Try to imagine as well as you can, or try to hear yourself yelling stop very loudly.

Keep practicing until you can get it as clear and as loud as possible. Then open your eyes." When the client opens his or her eyes, the therapist asks whether the imagery was sufficiently clear and loud and able to evoke a jolt. If the client reports some problem, he or she is asked to practice again. If there is still a problem, the client is encouraged to yell "stop" out loud several times and then to rehearse the technique once more with the particular target thought. If, after some repetition, good auditory imagery still has not been obtained, the client may be asked to imagine seeing the word "stop" in red letters, while saying the word to himself or herself. Generally, after some practice, clients do not report any problems with imagery.

In ensuing trials, client and therapist alternate interruptions of the thought for approximately ten minutes (amounting to about twenty trials) until the client indicates that he or she has learned the procedure. At the end of the session, the client is instructed to rehearse the procedure at specified times during the day (two or three blocks of ten to twenty trials apiece) and whenever there is any spontaneous occurrence of the thoughts discussed during the assessment phase. In order to prevent discouragement if the thoughts recur, the therapist points out that there is more value in repeating "stop" than in entertaining the thought. Clients are reminded that with the use of TS, the target thought will occur less and less frequently, until it finally disappears altogether. A weekly check is made of the frequency of practice, the specific thought that occurred, and any failures experienced with the TS practice.

During each subsequent therapy session, five to ten minutes a week are allotted to rehearsal of the TS procedure. This time allotment may be increased or decreased, depending on the amount of practice by the client and on the client's progress. When the client is first learning the procedure, he or she is told to interrupt the thought only at its initiation (e.g., "Signal when you *begin* to think the thought"). Subsequent trials deal with the thought in various stages nearing completion. (For example: "Signal when you arrive at the word ________.") Finally, other trials are presented in which the thought sequence is interrupted on a random basis instead of at each occurrence.

## Cognitive Strategies

### *Self-Talk*

The procedures suggested by Albert Ellis (1970) will be an appropriate place to start our discussion of cognitive techniques. Ellis has succinctly summarized his views as follows:

> Rational-emotive psychotherapy is a comprehensive approach to psychological treatment that deals not only with the emotional and behavioral aspects of human disturbance, but places a great deal of

> stress on its thinking component. Human beings are exceptionally complex, and there neither seems to be any simple way in which they become "emotionally disturbed," nor is there a single way in which they can be helped to be less self-defeating. Their psychological problems arise from their misperceptions and mistaken cognitions about what they perceive; from their emotional underreactions or overreactions to normal and unusual stimuli; and from their habitually dysfunctional behavior patterns, which enable them to keep repeating nonadjustive responses even when they know that they are behaving poorly. (p. 2)

Maladaptive feelings and actions are seen as the result of maladaptive or "irrational" thoughts. The thrust of the therapy is to demonstrate to the patient that the "crazy," "sick," or "maladaptive" consequences of thoughts are a result of false, irrational, or mistaken beliefs or self-talk and not of the actions or experiences that preceded them.

There are many illogical statements that Ellis feels are very commonplace in our culture. Once you are aware of what those self-defeating, illogical, and "internalized self-talks" are, you can put your finger on a few central beliefs that your patient brings to therapy. Below is a list of some of the core irrational beliefs that are held to be at the root of most emotional disturbance. Each is followed by a more reasonable substitute that the therapist attempts to get the patient to accept:

- The idea that it is a dire necessity for an adult to be loved by everyone for everything he or she does—instead of concentrating on one's own self-respect, on winning approval for practical purposes, and on loving rather than on being loved.

- The idea that human misery is externally caused and is forced on one by outside people and events—instead of the idea that emotional disturbance is caused by the *view* one takes of conditions.

- The idea that if something is or may be dangerous or fearsome one should be terribly upset about it—instead of the idea that one would do better to frankly face it and render it nondangerous or, when that is not possible, accept the inevitable.

- The idea that because something once strongly affected one's life, it should indefinitely affect it—instead of the idea that one can learn from one's past experiences but not be overly attached to or prejudiced by them.

- The idea that human happiness can be achieved by inertia and inaction—instead of the idea that humans tend to be happiest when they are vitally absorbed in creative pursuits, or when they are devoting themselves to people or projects outside themselves.

The cognitive technique of focusing patients or clients on their self-talk, the "soft internal whispers" that often occur prior to their actions, is a valuable contribution to any therapist's armamentarium regardless of theoretical orientation.

Meichenbaum (1977) and Beck et al. (1979) have both elaborated on the idea that a patient's self-talk "can get them in trouble." Statements people say to themselves, irrational or otherwise, will determine what they do. These statements are based on idiosyncratic experiences and result in a number of faulty ideas regarding their condition.

As with behavior therapy, the patient is trained to observe and record, but thoughts rather than behaviors. Beck (1979) presents the following illustration of how this occurs, while working with a 43-year-old depressed patient:

Therapist: The way a person thinks about or interprets events affects how he feels and behaves. For example, say he was home alone one night and heard a crash in another room. If he thinks, "There's a burglar in the room," how do you think he would feel?

Patient: Very anxious, terrified.

T: And how might he behave?

P: He might try to hide or if he was smart he would phone the police.

T: Okay, so in response to a thought that a burglar made the noise, the person would probably feel anxious and behave in such a way as to protect himself. Now, let's say he heard the same noise and thought, "The windows have been left open and the wind has caused something to fall over." How would he feel?

P: Well, he wouldn't be afraid. He might be sad if he thought something valuable was broken or he might be annoyed that one of the kids left the window open.

T: And would his behavior be different following this thought?

P: Sure, he would probably go and see what the problem was. He certainly wouldn't phone the police.

T: Okay. Now, what this example shows us is that there are usually a number of ways in which you can interpret a situation. Also, the way you interpret the situation affects your feelings and behavior. (pp. 147–149)

*Cognitive Restructuring*

Cognitive restructuring encompasses a series of techniques aimed at modifying thinking and reasoning. We've already discussed Ellis's view regarding the irrational belief system patients tenaciously hold. Beck (1979) focuses on the patient's distorted thought patterns. Distortions include:

- arbitrary inferences not supported by evidence
- magnification and exaggeration of the significance of an event
- cognitive deficiency or disregard for an important element in a situation
- dichotomous reasoning or seeing things as either black or white (good or bad, right or wrong, with no in-betweens)
- overgeneralization from a single incident

Clients are taught to identify these distortions through semantic and behavioral techniques. The therapist then challenges the "silent assumptions" underlying clients' attitudes and conceptions by demonstrating the clients' unrealistic interpretations of their experiences. The clients then collaborate in observing and analyzing their own experiences.

*Reframing and Restructuring*

Reframing and restructuring are yet other techniques cognitive therapists use when combating the mistaken notions their patients have regarding themselves. Reframing allows the patient to make an alteration in "the conceptual and/or emotional setting or viewpoint in relation to which a situation is experienced and to place it in another frame which fits the facts of the same concrete situation equally well or even better, merely changing its entire meaning." (Watzlawick et al., 1974, p. 12) Thus, feelings, actions, and their consequences are changed by changing attributed meanings.

Family therapists such as Satir (1967) and Minuchin and Fishman (1981) are especially adept at exploring the relationship within the therapy session with the major aim of helping families restructure their experiences. Unlike the analytically oriented therapist who interprets and analyzes the relationship, or the behaviorally oriented therapist who uses the relationship to entice the patient to act differently, the cognitive therapist attempts to restructure the patient's thoughts by focusing on what occurs in the relationship.

> A child spills crayons and walks away, a father yells, the child starts to pick up and walks away . . . . the father ignores the child, feeling satisfied that he did his job; the mother walks near the child and softly reminds the child that the job has not been finished . . . . the child completes the job.

Later a discussion of the incident reveals that both parents identify father as the competent, constructive influence on the family while mother is seen as soft and inefficient in her ability to control the child. Her thinking regarding her ability to control the child will be the focus of the intervention, rather than helping her learn "new" ways to "discipline."

Mahoney (1974) advocates providing patients with mnemonic aids to help when they are learning to cognitively restructure their experiences. For example, Mahoney has used the label *ADAPT* to remind patients of a restructuring sequence. Each letter stands for a particular sequence in the process:

> **A** *Acknowledge* the sensation of distress (anxiety, depression, anger),
>
> **D** *Discriminate* the private events (both thoughts and images) which have just occurred (i.e., do a "covert instant replay"),
>
> **A** *Assess* the logical bases and adaptive functions of your images and self-statements,
>
> **P** *Present* alternatives (i.e., generate private monologues or imagery of more appropriate, coping content) and then,
>
> **T** *Think* praise (!) (i.e., reward yourself for having executed the entire sequence). (p 156)

## SUMMARY

The dynamic and cognitive–behavioral approaches to intervention were described and contrasted in this chapter. The dynamic approach affords special emphasis to the patient/therapist relationship while the cognitive–behavioral approach pays more attention to techniques and principles of intervention. These two major approaches are by no means mutually exclusive, and clinicians in independent practice are wise to fit their interventions to the client's needs rather than try to force the client to fit a specialized theory.

Chapter 11

# On Being an Expert Witness

# 11

The interplay between the legal and mental health professions was at one time considered an arcane subject. When a mental health professional was consulted for an "expert opinion," it was usually a psychiatrist being asked to testify to the "sanity" or "insanity" of a person standing trial for murder.

A confluence of events has emerged to change the texture of psycholegal activities. Violence and disruption of the social environment, penal reform emphasizing rehabilitation rather than revenge and punishment, the rise of divorce with the ensuing problems of custody of the children, the emerging juvenile justice system, the more frequent use of alcohol and drugs, and the greater acceptance of mental health services by the public at large, are some of the factors that have contributed to the need for both lawyers and mental health practitioners to work collaboratively if they are to provide the best service to the client.

An informal survey of a dozen independent mental health practitioners in the Rochester area revealed that on the average they had four contacts a year with the legal system. Of the approximately 40 incidents only one involved murder; the rest were minor criminal issues such as mental state while driving, drug-related problems, juvenile delinquency, and civil actions surrounding divorce and custody.

It is now not uncommon for psychologists, social workers, guidance counselors, psychotherapists, as well as psychiatrists to be called to the witness stand to testify as expert witnesses.

Caught up in the advocacy process, the expert witness is either for or against the attorney's client. However, according to Brodsky and Robey (1972), the ideal role of the mental health expert witness "is that of a detached, thoroughly neutral individual who simply and informatively presents the true facts as he sees them: the undesirable role is that of a partisan seeking to undermine the opponent, acting deceptively to present 'his' case more favorably and behaving in a variety of unethical, inappropriate ways for reasons of greed, maladjustment, or personal aggrandizement" (p. 173).

The position that the mental health professional should strive to be an impartial witness free from prejudice and not act as an advocate for either side can be found in a number of discussions of psychiatric testimony (Bromberg, 1979; MacDonald, 1969; and Slovenko, 1973). However, called upon as an expert witness you have to be prepared for a different set of rules and roles than those learned as a student or practiced in the usual settings in which you find yourself acting as an expert, such as consulting rooms, schools, or hospitals.

This chapter will familiarize the clinician with the legal proceedings in which he or she might have occasion to participate as an expert witness. The major aim will be to help make you more comfortable and effective as a witness in legal proceedings, by informing you of what is expected of you in a court of law. Mental health practitioners receive little if any formal training in this area and often do not possess even a knowledgeable vocabulary with which to communicate. Liebenson and Wepman (1964) have provided a list of common legal terms with which mental health practitioners should become familiar. This list is from their book, *The Psychologist as Expert Witness,* and is reproduced below with permission of their publisher.

## GLOSSARY OF LEGAL TERMS

**Admission**—The confession or voluntary acknowledgment made by a party to a civil action either orally, in writing, or by his action, as to the existence or truth of certain facts.

**Answer**—The document filed by the defendant in answer to the charges in the complaint, in which he admits or denies the allegations.

**Burden of Proof**—That degree of proof necessary to prove the issues in civil or criminal proceedings. In civil cases the burden of proof is to prove the issue by preponderance or greater weight of evidence. In a criminal action the state is required to prove its case beyond a reasonable doubt.

**Civil Action**—An action which is instituted to recover for the infraction of a private or civil right and in most instances recovery is based upon the compensation for the breach of the right. Any action which is not criminal is said to be a civil action.

**Complaint or Declaration**—The document filed in court at the beginning of a lawsuit, containing the charges against the defendant. The complaint notifies the defendant of the wrongs alleged to have been committed by him and also notifies him of the amount of damages he is asked to pay.

**Confession**—The voluntary admission of a criminal act by a person who committed the crime or misdemeanor, to another of his own acts in the commission or participation which he had in a criminal act.

**Contract Action**—A lawsuit based upon the breach of an oral or written contract.

**Corpus Delicti**—Literally, the body of the offense. This is distinguished from the participation of any person in a crime. It applies in criminal law. The law requires proof of two propositions: one, that the criminal act was done, and two, that it was done by the person or persons charged. The corpus delicti is the proof that is necessary to prove that the act was done.

**Crime**—An act or omission prohibited by public law. Such public law to be considered a crime must be made for the protection of the public, and made punishable by the state in a judicial proceeding in its own name.

**Criminal Action**—An action which deals with the breach of crimes and offenses against the local, state, or federal government. The action is brought in the name of the people of the state rather than in an individual name.

**Criminal Information**—A criminal information is an accusation or complaint exhibited against a person for some criminal offense. It differs from an indictment in that it is not cast upon by a grand jury, but is the allegation of a public officer. An information, in most instances, applies to misdemeanors.

**Cross-Examination**—The sequence of questions asked the witness by the opposing attorney, after direct examination has been completed.

**Defendant**—The party being sued.

**Deposition for Discovery Purposes**—A procedure permitted in most states whereby an opposing attorney has the right to question any witness, under oath, before a notary public or other officer of the court, for the purpose of giving the opposing side information desired from the witness. Questions are asked by the opposing attorney as though the witness were on the witness stand and under cross-examination. This procedure is conducted before trial and aids the parties to the lawsuit in giving them a better understanding of the claims of the opposing side. The trial itself is simplified because most information is obtained during deposition.

**Deposition to Perpetuate Testimony**—A right given any party to the lawsuit to take the testimony of any witness with the same effect as though the witness were in court and testifying from the witness stand. This procedure is permitted only in cases in which the witness lives outside the boundaries of the court's power, or the witness is too ill to come to court. Testimony is usually taken before the trial starts. The witness is asked questions by both counsels as though he were in court. The testimony is recorded and read at the trial. This testimony has the same weight and value as any other evidence presented. Practically speaking, such testimony should be avoided when possible, as it is more effective for the jury and court to see and hear the witness.

**Direct Examination**—The sequence of questions asked of a witness by the attorney who has called him to the witness stand for his side of the case.

**Evidence**—All testimony adduced from witnesses on the witness stand, which is not stricken from the record by the judge. It also includes all documents, papers, photographs and x-rays which the judge allows to be considered.

**Felony**—A crime which is punishable by prison sentence of more than one year duration.

**Homicide**—The killing of a human being.

**Impeachment**—A technique of questioning by the opposing attorney during cross-examination to discredit testimony by demonstrating that the witness has made previous oral or written statements contradictory to a major part of his testimony on the witness stand.

**Indictment**—A written accusation against one or more persons naming them for the breach of a crime. The indictment must be presented by a grand jury which has been legally invoked. They must hear evidence under oath and vote on such indictment before it becomes a legal document. An assent of at least twelve grand jurors is necessary.

**Misdemeanor**—A minor offense generally punishable by a sentence under one year in duration.

**Objection**—The expression used by an attorney to the judge to express his opinion that a rule of evidence has been infracted by the opposing side.

**Objection Overruled**—The expression used by the judge to signify that the objection is without legal basis.

**Objection Sustained**—The expression used by the judge to indicate that the objection made was good, and that the judge has ruled with the party making the objection.

**Plaintiff**—The party bringing the lawsuit.

**Recross-Examination**—The sequence of questions following redirect examination, asked by the attorney who questioned on direct examination. This is to elaborate or clarify answers made by the witness during cross-examination.

**Subpoena**—An order issued by the court requiring a person or corporation to bring specified records to court at a particular time and place, for use during a case on trial.

**Summons**—The official notice served upon the defendant notifying him of the lawsuit. A summons must be served before the defendant is "legally" before the court. Many states have provisions in their laws for other means of notifying the defendant of the lawsuit. Such provisions pertain to instances in which substituted service is permitted if it is not possible to give the summons to the defendant personally.

**Tort Action**—A civil action for the breach of a private or civil wrong or injury other than a contract.

**Undue Influence**—Any improper constraint or form of persuasion whereby the will of another is overpowered, and the party is induced to act otherwise than he would have done. Some courts hold this synonymous with the word "duress."

**Witness**—The party testifying on the witness stand.

## PRETRIAL PREPARATION FOR A COURT HEARING

The second step in the mental health practitioner's education for becoming a more effective expert witness may be delineated as the pretrial phase. Brodsky and Robey (1974) have enumerated a number of "harmful" attitudes and behaviors that witnesses unfamiliar with legal procedures bring with them to the courtroom. Some attitudes and behaviors that can spell disaster for the mental health practitioner whose reputation is on the line in public display follow:

- little or no relevant training
- poor record keeping in terms of important dates, times, pre- and postoccurrences
- reaction to a subpoena with fear and distress
- lack of awareness of legal position
- preparation as if attending a professional conference
- minimal if any pretrial contact with lawyer

Furthermore, poor preparation is likely to lead to poor, ineffective testimony, and possible disastrous effects for the practitioner especially during cross-examination. Negative experiences will in turn affect the practitioner's willingness to become involved with court cases, or even cases that hint of legal involvement in the future. They can also influence how much the client will be billed.

Independent practitioners who are novices regarding mental health legal activities seem to unrealistically over- or undercharge for their services in comparison with their customary fee. It is certainly reasonable to expect a higher fee for your services when called upon as an expert witness; however, the fee charged should be based on your *regular* hourly fee, and the time spent in:

- evaluation of the client
- interpreting and reporting the information
- courtroom time
- preparation time including pretrial conferences with lawyer

As you conduct your practice and prepare specifically for your testimony on the witness stand, keep the following points in mind:

- Careful preparation is the key to effective testimony. As a rule, whenever a case may involve a legal proceeding, you should record your findings in detail. Clearly record the dates and clearly document your observations and impressions.
- Your clinical records will probably be subpoenaed. Carefully review them and expect careful examination and cross-examination based on this information.
- Have as many communications with the attorney before the trial as you deem necessary. You should discuss the types of questions that will be asked of you, and you can even "role play" a few questions and answers with the attorney.

## THE WITNESS STAND

### Direct Examination

Expect to feel nervous while waiting to testify. Something that helps with the "waiting anxiety" is to review your notes and consider the main points you plan to establish. Spontaneous responses are more believable and thus you should neither "memorize your testimony" nor plan to extensively refer to your notes on the witness stand.

You can also expect a surge of anxiety when called into the courtroom to present your testimony and especially as judge and lawyers watch you enter. Try not to avoid their glance and remember that they view every witness who enters the courtroom in a similar manner.

The first person who will respond to you will be the bailiff who will "swear you in." Then—you're on! Some common symptoms of nervousness as you get ready to answer the first question are (1) perceptual problems in the courtroom, especially of sight, (2) lowering of the voice, (3) slumping in the witness chair, (4) speaking rapidly, (5) speaking in a monotone, and (6) inability to recognize anyone in the courtroom.

To overcome these possible symptoms, Shrybman and Halpern (1979) suggest the following:

Sit with your back straight, taking care not to allow your shoulders to slump or your body to slide down in the chair. Start out straight and you have a better chance of staying that way; a curled up witness may not make as good an impression on the judge as an erect witness.

Look around the room to orient yourself. Look at the rear of the room and the walls you can see without turning around.

Most witnesses tend to lower their voices and speak a little faster. You can help yourself relax and make a better appearance by speaking a little louder and slower than you feel is necessary. Try especially to avoid long pauses.

The testimony brought out in the original questioning by the attorney who asks you to testify is called direct evidence. When asked to provide evidence by your attorney establishing the nature, extent, and seriousness of the disorders in the client, or your opinion as to the cause of the disorders, you are providing the court with direct evidence. You are allowed to use your records or any other notes while testifying. Remember, the opposing attorney has the right during cross-examination to see such reports and notes and ask questions based on information in them.

Shrybman and Halpern (1979) have suggested a number of key principles the clinician should be aware of before testifying:

1. If you do not understand the question, have it repeated. Never guess at what a question means. If you do not know the answer to a question, say so. Do not guess at answers; answer only questions asked; do not volunteer answers.
2. If you are asked to give a yes or no answer and feel that such an answer would be misleading without an explanation, ask the judge to allow you to explain the answer properly, or indicate to your attorney that you want to explain that answer. In any case, never get angry or defensive with the defense attorney.
3. Be exact in your testimony. For example, say "1 P.M." instead of "around noon," or "three occasions" instead of "numerous occasions."
4. Your responses to questions must be spoken. Such nonverbal communications as nodding, shaking, or gesturing your head will not be acceptable to the court. Do not volunteer information and only answer the questions asked.

   You must listen to each question so you know what information is appropriate. For example:

   Q. You stated that you are a licensed clinical psychologist. Where did you get your training?

That means formal schooling in psychology—not the elementary and high schools you attended or the degrees you received that do not relate to your professional skills.

Q. What did you and Thomas Jones talk about during your first interview?

Give the time, date, and place of the conversation; then tell the substance of the conversation or topics discussed.

Q. How is a psychologist different from a psychiatrist?

A. A psychiatrist is a physician who specializes in treating diseases of the mind. A psychiatrist is licensed to dispense medication and is qualified by law to perform the functions of a medical doctor. A psychologist is a Ph.D. who determines an individual's current behavior, attitudes, and feelings from psychological tests administered. Psychology is a separate discipline from medicine and is regulated by different procedures and practices.

When on the witness stand, be alert and aware of the kind of response desired. Direct examination, questions asked by the attorney who requested you to testify, usually calls for narrative responses; cross-examination, questions asked by the opposing attorney, most often can be answered with a "yes" or "no."

5. Do not jump the gun when answering questions, but let your attorney develop your testimony.

   Q. Do you remember an interview with Alice White on Wednesday, May 15, at 11 A.M.?

   The best response is "Yes" or "No." In the next question, the attorney may ask you to narrate the substance of the interview. The purpose of the first question is to prepare a foundation before introducing the significant part of your testimony.

6. Take care to explain all clinical terms so that the judge, attorneys, and jury are able to understand your testimony. Check with the attorney who is calling you as a witness to identify some of the technical phrases that may come up during your testimony. The following is a partial listing of terms you might have to use while testifying. How would you explain them?

   - subdural hematoma
   - childhood adjustment reaction
   - psychosis
   - manic-depressive
   - neurosis
   - phobia
   - schizophrenia
   - involutional

- delusional thinking
- psychiatric social worker
- milieu therapy
- partial hospitalization program
- learning disability
- hyperactive
- an acute episode
- failure to thrive
- mental illness
- multidisciplinary evaluation
- labile
- suicidal ideation
- passive-aggressive behavior
- character disorder
- reaction formation
- depression
- regression
- acting-out behavior
- withdrawn behavior
- autisticlike manifestations
- social history
- developmentally disabled

7. Keep in mind that your major responsibility as a witness is to impart information. Your job is not to "win" the case for the client; that is the attorney's role. Although you are part of an advocacy process, and you are being paid by the client, keep your testimony honest and maintain your credibility as an expert witness.

## The Expert Witness

Unlike most witnesses who can testify only about those facts they know personally, not about what others have said to them, the expert witness can give testimony from other sources. In such cases admissible evidence will be given through the use of a hypothetical question. Statements made to you by parents and children in a neglect case usually are also admissible as evidence.

The expert witness is allowed to give opinions in areas related to his or her expertise, whereas most witnesses are allowed to testify only as to factual matters—what *they* have seen, heard, or felt. They are not allowed to give their opinions about what these facts mean. Once you qualify as an expert witness in mental health areas, you are allowed to express your opinions in order to help the judge or hearing officer decide the case. For example, a social worker may qualify as an expert witness as to the behavior patterns of the parents or child.

In order to qualify as an expert, you will be asked to show how you are different from the ordinary witness and that you possess special knowledge and experience with regard to issues before the court. You can be expected to be asked questions regarding your education, years of experience, type of profession and subspecialty, professional affiliations, honorary societies, publications, and writings in your general area, or on the matter before the court.

A mistake is often made by witnesses when answering opinion questions. The question is "Do you have an opinion . . . ?" concerning an aspect of the case. At the end of the question the witness usually gives his or her opinion, which is a mistake. The correct answer to this question is "I do have an opinion." After this answer, the next question will be "What is your opinion?" Then the witness should state the opinion. When the expert answers the first question by giving an opinion there usually is an objection, which is sustained by the court because the question asks if the witness has an opinion. When the court sustains the objection, the witness may become confused and perhaps never get to answer the question.

After hearing the opinion, the attorney will ask the expert "What are the reasons for your opinion?" This is when all the preparation pays off and you have your opportunity to shine. It is important for you to have your reasons organized in your mind so that your answer to the question will be:

- clear
- concise
- explained in lay language
- presented in logical sequence

The hypothetical question, used in both criminal and civil cases, is another opinion question expert witnesses are expected to answer. In this instance you are only required to state your opinion based upon a reasonable degree of certainty. Liebenson and Wepman (1964) suggest that the mental health practitioner adopt the following attitude when answering hypothetical questions:

> These people who have to pass upon this case have no basis for a decision as to the technical or scientific issues unless I help them with my knowledge and experience based upon the facts of this case. Of course, I will give my opinions to what may reasonably have caused this condition, or whatever could possibly result from

> the particular facts within my knowledge. In other words, I am similar to a teacher trying to help my students understand a new subject matter. In this respect, my thinking has to be more liberal and my interpretation of the facts as to the unknown much broader than usual. I also understand that once this case is decided, neither party can ask that the jury change its decision. Basically, this should be the attitude of the expert witness. (p. 127)

**Cross-Examination**

Cross-examination is usually the most difficult part of testifying. The key to effective performance during cross-examination is adequate preparation, remembering to remain calm, and not become defensive, angry, or condescending. Such attitudes will diminish your credibility with the judge or jury and will detract from your ability to respond competently to the questions asked.

During cross-examinations, clinicians are tripped up on the "degree of certainty" with which they are able to testify about a particular condition. Remember, often you are not in a position to be 100 percent certain of the condition, but can provide reasons why, in your best professional judgment, you believe the current condition is influencing the patient's actions.

Another strategy often used is to "discredit" your expertise by closely questioning you on your previous experience with these types of cases, with the aim of showing that you are not specifically experienced in the particular area. This strategy is principally designed to upset you.

The cross-examiner may attempt to suggest details to you that you do not remember and that you did not state on direct examination. Do not follow the cross-examiner's leading question into an answer. For example, the cross-examiner may present a question in such a way that it seems imminently logical. However, if that is not what you remember, do not agree with the cross-examiner. Your suggestibility may cause you to change your answers without realizing it. Consider this exchange:

Q. In your report you stated that Billy could not walk to school because he lives too far from the school, didn't you?

You the witness think "Well, I remember there was concern about walking or driving to school. I don't remember specifically . . . but that is a good reason to ride the bus. I'll say yes."

A. Yes.

In fact, Billy only lives three blocks from the school. This discrepancy will be argued by the cross-examiner as impeaching your credibility.

Especially during cross-examination, if you do not understand a question, ask that it be repeated or rephrased; and do not volunteer information that can give the opposing attorney more ammunition to confuse you.

Be alert to compound questions and respond to each part separately. For example:

Q. Is it true that Mr. Brown stormed out of your office in a rage after your last appointment?

A. There are two parts to that question, and each part has a different answer. Mr. Brown did leave my office very angry, but we spoke briefly in my waiting room and he returned to my inner office where we resumed our meeting. When he left he was considerably calmer.

Never begin an answer to a compound question with "yes" because the attorney may cut you short and not allow you to complete your response, thus giving an erroneous impression of your actions.

When the opposing attorney ends a question with a "yes" or "no," do not feel obliged to answer the question in that manner. Start your answer with something like "Well, that needs some explaining." Even if the attorney objects, your position is stated and the attorney for your client will give you a chance to clarify your answer on redirect examination.

It is acceptable to be paid for your services as an expert witness. If questioned about this during cross-examination, feel free to state the fee you are being paid. Remember, lay witnesses receive statutory per diem allowances.

## THE LEGAL SYSTEM

Being familiar with the legal "ins and outs" of the judicial legal system will go a long way to making your day in court less taxing and add to your credibility as an expert witness.

You may be called as a witness to testify in "criminal" or "civil" cases. In a criminal case, the issue centers around a breach of some local, state, or federal law. A civil case involves a lawsuit by one person or persons against another person or persons for losses, injuries, or damages suffered as the result of another's acts. "Smith v. Brown" is an example of a civil action, whereas "People of the United States v. Franks" is an example of a criminal act alleged against the federal government.

The following material is intended for the mental health practitioner who may become involved with family and children's issues; however, for the most part, the information presented is applicable to all mental health clinicians.

### The Functions of Criminal Courts

Criminal courts have the following functions:

- to determine the guilt or innocence of the accused
- if the accused is found guilty, to determine appropriate punishment
- to mandate social services (as with terms of probation)
- to protect the constitutional rights of parents and children

### The Authority of Criminal Courts

Criminal courts have jurisdiction over the adult accused of committing a crime. The court in a criminal proceeding has no authority to make orders concerning a child unless special circumstances are met, as when an adolescent is accused of a crime such as murder.

The court may fine or imprison a defendant convicted of a crime. The criminal court may also place the defendant on probation. Probation is usually granted conditionally, that is, the defendant must do certain things, such as seek employment or obtain therapy or counseling, or abstain from doing other things, such as beating his wife.

### Procedures of Criminal Courts

Criminal prosecutions are initiated by the police department that arrests the defendant and in most cases refers the case to the county prosecutor. The prosecutor's office makes a separate discretionary decision as to whether the case will be prosecuted.

Criminal prosecutions of child abuse and neglect cases are handled in the same manner as other criminal prosecutions. The defendant is entitled to an attorney and to a jury trial if requested.

### The Juvenile Courts

Juvenile courts, or family courts, as they are called in many states, are where neglect, custody, abuse, and delinquency cases are heard. Juvenile courts work closely with social service agencies to formulate treatment plans designed to protect the child and improve the family situation with the primary aim of preserving the family system. Rehabilitation rather than punishment is of primary concern. In addition, the family court reviews the decisions of social service agencies and protects the constitutional rights of parents and children.

The juvenile court has jurisdiction over minors and is involved in delinquency cases (alleged criminal conduct by a minor) or in dependency cases (minors allegedly abused or neglected by their parents or other caretakers). Since the juvenile court has no jurisdiction over the parents in an abuse or neglect case, the court cannot directly enforce its orders against the parents of a child by fines, imprisonment, or threats of either. The juvenile court has leverage against parents only by its power over the child. For example, after finding that a child has been neglected, the juvenile court can order the child to remain in the home with the parents on the provision that the family become involved in psychotherapy. If the parents fail to comply, the court can order the child removed from the home and placed in a foster home or other care setting. When the court takes jurisdiction over a child, the court can

- order the child placed in his or her home under the supervision of the juvenile court probation department or the department of social services
- order the child placed with relatives, if they are able and willing to care for the child
- order the child placed in a foster home, group home, or institutional home

It is the responsibility of the juvenile court to guarantee that both parents and child have the opportunity for a fair and impartial hearing in a court of law. During the 1970s, family court became increasingly more formal and more strict in adhering to rules of evidence and procedure. This has led to greater importance of the role of the attorneys in family court hearings.

*Proceedings*

Shrybman and Halpern (1979) have summarized the hearing process in juvenile court:

> A juvenile court abuse and neglect case can be initiated by the filing of a petition (written complaint) in the juvenile court alleging that a child (or children) has been abused or neglected. The petition may be written and filed by the county attorney, the juvenile probation officer and/or a county social worker according to state law and local court procedures. (In a few states, anyone can can file a petition alleging that a child is abused or neglected.)
>
> In emergency situations where there is imminent danger to the child in remaining with the parent(s), the child may be removed from the custody of its parent(s) and placed in protective custody

pending the outcome of a juvenile court proceeding. This decision may be made by the police, juvenile probation, the juvenile court, child protective services and/or a physician, depending on state law. Whenever a child is placed in protective custody, a petition must be filed in the juvenile court, usually within 24 to 48 hours, and a hearing must be held soon thereafter (usually within 48 to 72 hours, depending on state law), to allow a judge to review the decision.

There has to be an evidentiary trial in which the state must prove to a judge that a child is abused or neglected. Unless the parent(s) admits that he/she has neglected or abused the child, it will be necessary to call witnesses to substantiate the allegations of abuse or neglect. The adjudicatory hearing usually occurs from two to six weeks after the initial petition is filed. Because a dependency hearing is civil rather than criminal, the state need not prove abuse or neglect beyond a reasonable doubt, but only by a preponderance of the evidence, a somewhat lower standard of proof. This is called an adjudication hearing.

Child abuse and neglect proceedings are usually "bifurcated proceedings," meaning the decision as to what should be done with the abused or neglected child occurs in a separate hearing from that which determines whether the child is, in fact, abused or neglected. A dispositional hearing, which is analogous to the sentencing hearing in a criminal case, may occur on the same day as the adjudicatory hearing or be held on a separate day, sometimes weeks later. The dispositional hearing usually focuses on the recommendation made to the judge by the court social worker regarding the appropriate order for the child.

In some states, no review hearings will be held. In others, they will be an integral part of the hearing process. After a child has been declared dependent, the juvenile court retains jurisdiction over that child until the child reaches adulthood or until the dependency status is ended by the juvenile court. In order to measure the progress of the case and determine any need to modify its previous order, the juvenile court will hold periodic hearings to review the case. These are generally held every six months to a year. (pp. 7–8)

### *Key Participants*

The judge is the key person in the juvenile court process. He or she is responsible for ensuring that fair and proper court procedures are observed at all times. In addition, the judge decides whether the child is abused or neglected and is responsible for determining the appropriate plan.

In most juvenile courts, there will be a county attorney (district attorney, corporation counsel) whose job is to present the child abuse and neglect case to the court. At times, social workers or probation officers present the case in court without assistance of an attorney.

The parents can have an attorney representing their interests, which is to defend against the allegations of abuse or neglect at the adjudicatory hearing or avoid placing the child out of their home at a dispositional hearing.

An attorney can also be appointed for the child. The Federal Child Abuse and Neglect Prevention and Treatment Act of 1974 requires that a state appoint a guardian "ad litem" ("in a law suit") for the child in a child abuse and neglect proceeding if that state is to be eligible for federal funds for child abuse and neglect programs. (The Act does not specify that the guardian must be an attorney.) When this occurs, there are usually at least three attorneys involved in a hearing—attorneys for the state, the parents, and the child. The main aim of the child's attorney is to represent his or her best interests by making sure, whenever possible, that the child's views are heard. The child's attorney usually plays a key role at the disposition hearing in presenting a plan for the child's future placement.

Witnesses may also participate in juvenile court hearings. These can include the petitioner, representatives from child protective services, probation officers, police, social workers, physicians, teachers, nurses, relatives, the child, the parents, and any other individuals having relevant information. If necessary, subpoenas will be issued to compel the attendance of witnesses at the adjudicatory hearing.

### *Some Important Forensic Issues*

Initially, the court has to decide whether or not it has jurisdiction to act; that is, it must decide whether the individual before the court falls within a prescribed statutory classification. The following are some typical statutory classifications and dispositional alternatives that would be of special interest to mental health practitioners.

- *Child Abuse and Neglect*—A child is generally considered neglected when (1) the parent, guardian, or other custodian has abandoned or abused the child. There is not proper parental care, control, or subsistence, or education as required by law, or other care or control necessary for the child's physical, mental, or emotional health; and the deprivation is not the result of financial limitations. (2) The parent, guardian, or other custodian is incarcerated, hospitalized, or physically or mentally incapacitated and not able to provide proper care for the child.

The primary aim of the court is to preserve the family bond unless such preservation endangers the welfare of the child. Consequently, the court will attempt to arrange a disposition that permits the parents to maintain custody of their child unless such custody is harmful to the child. The judge can also order the families to seek medical, psychiatric, or other treatment services.

If the court finds that placement with the family is not possible, then relatives, other qualified individuals, or commitment to the Department of Social Services or other agency for foster placement will be necessary. When more than one child is involved, the court prefers to keep siblings together in order to preserve whatever family bonds remain, and to ease the transition to a foster home if that is the disposition.

It is important to know that unless neglected children are also found to be delinquent, they cannot be committed to, or confined in, an institution for delinquent children. The court can also free a child for adoption by termination of parental rights.

• *Persons in Need of Supervision (PINS)*—A Person in Need of Supervision is in need of care and supervision because he or she habitually truants himself or herself from school without justification or he or she is habitually disobedient of the reasonable and lawful commands of his or her parent, guardian, or other custodian, and is ungovernable.

These cases are usually troublesome matters, clinically as well as legally. When parents and social agencies are unable or unwilling to find a solution for a troubled or troublesome child, it is in society's interest to try, through its legal system, to *prevent* crime and delinquency via an attempt at rehabilitation rather than wait to punish its occurrence.

Family and juvenile court has at its disposal an array of social services, as well as traditional judicial remedies. Referral to court should not be used for children with discipline problems at home or who are having minor difficulties in school. Only when they are at risk of becoming a delinquent should this step be taken. The court has considerable leeway when fashioning a plan for disposition. Children may even be placed in facilities for delinquents if they have twice been adjudicated a PINS.

• *Juvenile Delinquency*—The juvenile court generally has jurisdiction over juveniles accused of committing a crime who are under the age of 18 years on the date of the commission of the act. Recent changes in the law (Guggenheim, 1979) have introduced some new exceptions to jurisdiction over children age 13 or older charged with murder, forceable rape, robbery while armed, first-degree burglary, or assault with intent to commit any of the above. Juveniles age 15 and over at the time of the offense who are charged with a felony may be transferred to the appropriate criminal division for trial, as well as juveniles age 16 or over who have previously been committed to an institution and are charged in a new delinquency petition with any offense.

The juvenile court's relationship to a child is a meld of providing for the "best interest of the child" along with protection of the community. The court can decide to dismiss a youth, that is, grant an outright dismissal of the charge. This motion might be considered where a minor offense is charged against a first offender and court supervision of the child would be necessary. A consent decree can also be granted by the court and may be entered if the child has not been previously adjudicated a delinquent by the court, or if such adjudication has been sealed (is not available to the court). Under a consent decree a juvenile is put on probation for up to six months without a finding of guilt. Thus, the court can provide supervision without stigmatization. After successful completion of the specific terms of the decree, the original petition is dismissed. If the conditions of the decree are violated, the original petition may be reinstated and the juvenile forced to stand trial.

• *Mental Illness Commitments*—A person who is believed to be mentally ill, and because of the illness is likely to injure himself or herself or other persons if allowed to remain at liberty, may be committed to an institution. The judicial hospitalization of a person begins by the filing of a petition by her or his spouse, parent, or legal guardian, by a physician, by a duly accredited officer or agent of the Department of Public Health, or by an officer authorized to make arrests.

If after a hearing the person is not found to be mentally ill or if mentally ill is not ill to the extent that he or she is likely to injure himself or herself or other persons, the court will immediately order his or her release. If the court finds, after the hearing, that the person is mentally ill, and because of the illness is likely to injure himself or herself or other persons if allowed to remain at liberty, the court can commit the person to a hospital.

• *Handicapped Children*—Under the Education for All Handicapped Children Act of 1977, PL 94-142, every handicapped child is entitled to a free appropriate public education. The following are considered handicapped conditions: mentally retarded, hard of hearing, deaf, orthopedically impaired, other health impaired, speech impaired, visually handicapped, seriously emotionally disturbed, or children with specific learning disabilities who by reason thereof require special education and related services. The court first has to decide if the child has a handicapping condition and then whether or not the child is in need of special education.

Special education, according to statutory definition, involves only instruction that is designed and directed to meet the unique needs of a handicapped child and, therefore, will not be the totality of his or her education. Remember, intervention with a child does not occur because he or she is specifically learning disabled, but because the child has a unique educational need that requires specially designed instruction. The Act also states:

> A written statement for each handicapped child be developed in any meeting by a representative of the local education agency or an

> intermediate educational unit who shall be qualified to provide, or supervise the provision of, specially designed instruction to meet the unique needs of handicapped children, the teacher, the parents or guardian of such child, and whenever appropriate, such child, which statement shall include (a) a statement of the present levels of educational performance of such child, (b) a statement of annual goals, including short-term instructional objectives, (c) a statement of the specific educational services to be provided to such child, and the extent to which such child will be able to participate in regular educational programs, (d) the projected date for initiation and anticipated duration of such services, and appropriate objective criteria and evaluation procedures and schedules for determining, on at least an annual basis, whether instructional objectives are being achieved. (PL 94-142, 1977)

• *Child Custody*—The divorce statutes in all states authorize the court to issue orders concerning the custody of children of the marriage, as an incident to the divorce. Temporary orders may be made pending the divorce action for the protection of the children and final order in the divorce decree itself. Custody orders may also be made after the divorce decree. Custody orders are always subject to modification upon a showing of change in circumstances. Custody of a child is awarded to promote the child's best interests.

Some factors that are considered are the child's wishes (where appropriate), the age and sex of the child, the parents' strength, the ability of the parent to care for and supervise the child, the remarriage of a parent and the willingness of the new spouse to accept the child, the physical conditions in which the child is to live, and the mental health of the parent as it affects his or her ability to parent. When more than one child is involved, courts usually say that the children should not be separated unless their welfare very clearly requires such a course.

## SUMMARY

Ladies and gentlemen of the reading audience, I would like to sum up the material presented in this chapter with a brief A.B.C. approach to being an effective expert witness.

A. Antecedents of a successful expert witness require preparation. Do have meetings with the attorney prior to your court hearing. Prepare your material for presentation and anticipate some possible cross-examination questions.

B. When you find yourself on the witness stand, try to keep these points in mind:

- Speak directly to the judge or jury in a language that is readily understandable to the lay public.
- In testifying on behalf of a client, try to educate the judge or jury while explaining your answers. Remember the teaching-oriented conferences discussed in Chapter 5.
- Try to avoid traps and pitfalls under cross-examination; do not be afraid to say "I do not know" or to concede minor points.
- Avoid becoming defensive, abrupt, or brusque; instead remain calm, courteous, and consistent while testifying.

C. Your effective courtroom behavior can, of course, be helpful to your client, but, just as important, it can establish your credibility and integrity with the forensic community in your town.

Chapter 12

# From Earning a Living to Living on Earnings

# 12

Unlike salaried clinicians who are provided fringe benefits in addition to salary, independent practitioners have to provide for their own "benefits." These include

- income protection
- health insurance
- life insurance
- retirement plans
- professional liability insurance (malpractice)

Insurance and pension plans are two time-honored approaches available to wise and prudent independent practitioners who have to provide for their own "fringe package." Individuals' circumstances and the types of risks they are exposed to vary, as do their needs for convenience, security, and protection. Of course, the advice of an expert will be required to tailor an individualized program for you.

The aim of this chapter, written with the advice and aid of Bernard Golden, Certified Life Underwriter (CLU), will be to familiarize the reader with a number of options available and consider some strategies for using current income to provide for those times when you want to cut back, consider retirement, or when you might find yourself incapacitated.

## PROTECTION

### Life Insurance

Basically, there are two types of life insurance policies available to the practitioner: term and whole life.

Term life insurance protects the insured for a specific period of time and is the least expensive form of life insurance available. Term insurance is usually available to members of professional organizations, such as the American Medical Association, National Association of Social Workers, or the American Psychological Association, at considerably lower rates than individual rates. For example, the American Psychological Association provides an insurance trust that sponsors group life insurance plans through Liberty Mutual of Boston with a broad range of insurance coverage packages. Rates are lower because the insurance is provided to a large number of individuals through one master group plan. Like all group insurance plans, if you leave the group, or the master group plan is terminated, your protection is also terminated. The flexibility of an individual insurance plan is traded for lower premiums. Term insurance also provides protection for your home or office building mortgage.

Whole life or equity life insurance is more costly insurance because it provides less life insurance for higher premiums. However, a whole life insurance policy builds up equity, which can be used to purchase additional insurance, pay for current premiums, borrow against at considerably lower interest rates, or contribute to a retirement program.

Such factors as the number and age of dependents, their ability to support themselves, the amount of premium one can afford, the number of other assets, other benefits survivors might receive, and the income needed to permit one's family to live in a particular life style are important considerations when determining life insurance needs. Often part-time private practitioners have some life insurance provided through their salaried position.

You may consider purchasing both types of life insurances, some on an individualized basis and some on a group basis through your professional organization. The options open to you are varied. A consultation with a trusted independent insurance agent can help you avoid many life insurance pitfalls.

## Income Protection

When self-employed clinicians become disabled, their expenses continue despite the loss of income. Salaried professionals' sick leave benefits provide protection for at least a limited time, usually two to four weeks. Some public agencies permit accruing sick time not used in a calendar year up to a specified maximum, usually 26 or 52 weeks.

Self-employed clinicians, however, can depend only on themselves to pay for expenses such as rent, food, and clothing if their income has stopped. Savings, which will be needed for such expenses, expire very rapidly and if you are still unable to work the result is much hardship for yourself and your family.

Disability insurance is very costly insurance but highly desirable for the part-time, and virtually mandatory for the full-time, independent practitioner. Two factors determine the premiums:

1. the waiting period before receiving benefits
2. income to be received

Group policies that can be obtained through professional organizations such as The National Association of Social Workers or the American Psychological Association cost considerably less than income protection insurance taken out on an individual basis. Waiting periods vary and insurance can be obtained after a waiting period of one week or one month or one year. Benefits that begin without a waiting period are extremely expensive. A good strategy is to set aside a sum of money equivalent to that which you would earn during the waiting period. The type of plan you choose will depend on the weekly benefit you desire, the amount of coverage you already have, and your salary.

A significant portion of income received when one is ill or disabled is tax free and thus you will need less total gross income than you normally earn.

Most income protection plans also provide benefits for death or dismemberment. However, the benefits are usually quite conservative as this protection is not the primary purpose of income protection insurance. If your practice involves much travel or if you desire higher insurance coverage for death or dismemberment, separate insurance against these hazards should be considered.

**Medical Insurance**

Most of us take for granted medical insurance provided by Blue Cross and Blue Shield or similar policies underwritten by other companies to provide protection against the high cost of hospital and related medical services. Plans that cover the costs of medical, dental, and mental health services related to illness; plans that pay for the usual "everyday" medical expenses in addition to illness; and even protection designed to take over where the regular medical insurance policies leave off are available. Drug, X-ray, and eyeglass riders can also be added for an additional cost.

If married, you may be covered by a family medical plan provided by your spouse's employer. Such a plan may be fully or partially paid for by the employer.

As with other insurance plans discussed, group rates are considerably less expensive than individual rates. If you are a solo practitioner and consult to a group, consider buying your medical coverage through the group. If this is not feasible, you can combine an individual health insurance plan for "short"-term protection with a group "major medical" insurance program designed to take over where your basic plan leaves off. Such major medical plans are usually sponsored by major professional organizations and come with a variety of deductible amounts similar to automobile insurance.

For example, the American Psychological Association through the insurance trust and in conjunction with Liberty Mutual of Boston has made available to members a group major medical plan. All members of the APA are eligible to join the plan, but charges for pre-existing conditions, that is, conditions for which you were treated within six months before the effective date of insurance, are not covered. If, however, there is no charge for such pre-existing conditions for six consecutive months, then these conditions are also covered by the policy.

The premiums are determined by the size of the deductible ($500 or $1,000), the age of the member, and the type of contract (member; member and spouse; member and children; or member, spouse, and children). The premiums can range from less than $30 a year for a single, 30-year-old with a $1,000 deductible to over $300 for a 60-year-old married member with children.

## Professional Liability or Malpractice Insurance

I once asked an attorney if he thought I could sue and he replied, "You can always sue. Whether you'll win is another matter." Mental health facilities such as community mental health centers, psychiatric hospitals, child guidance clinics, and family service centers routinely insure their staff members against the risk of malpractice. The relatively low premium for nonmedical practitioners as contrasted with physicians reflects the small number of successful claims brought against nonmedical mental health practitioners.

Lewin (1978) reports that there were about 100 suits brought against psychologists between the ten-year period from 1961 to 1971; however, since then there have been almost 50 suits a year. It is not inconceivable for a patient to be awarded in excess of $100,000 if successful. Legal fees can run as high as $10,000. Malpractice insurance is one type of insurance that is a necessity.

Fortunately, most professional organizations have made arrangements through insurance underwriters to provide professional liability insurance to their members at a very modest cost. For less than $100.00 the nonmedical clinician can obtain malpractice insurance for $500,000 of aggregate claims in any one year. The American Professional Agency, Inc., 95 Broadway, Amityville, NY 11701, is a major provider of such insurance and can supply you with specific information regarding premiums and coverages.

Of course, prevention is the best protection when it comes to malpractice suits. The following guidelines are extremely important:

- Provide clinical coverage when on extended vacation. Even if away from the office for a few days, you are *legally* and clinically responsible for the practice.
- Document your sessions and decisions. This can work for you, especially when suicide is an issue (see Chapter 3).
- Physical contact, either assault or sexual intimacies, is, of course, unethical and insurance companies will be unlikely to pay for judgments awarded due to these charges.
- Discuss your plan of treatment with the client (see Chapter 3) and be sure not to release any information without the client's consent (or parents' consent in the case of a minor).

## RETIREMENT

Sheltering current income has become a major preoccupation of practitioners planning for their retirement. With tax sheltering the total amount of your permissible contribution is deducted from your taxable income. You pay no income tax on that amount. In a sense the federal government is underwriting a portion of your retirement program. If you are in the 40 percent tax bracket and are able to put $4,000 into your retirement plan, the government is actually contributing $1,600 and you are paying $2,400. The $1,600 is the amount you would otherwise be paying in taxes.

Furthermore, there is no current tax on the money generated by your investment. This enables your investment to be compounded and grow at an accelerated rate. Tax-deferred plans, unlike taxable investments or savings accounts, where you pay taxes on dividends and interest every year, require you to pay no taxes on income until you begin withdrawing funds. This usually occurs when you are in a lower tax bracket. For example, if you invested $2,000 for 10 years at 10 percent interest you would have $13,277 plus all the funds where taxable at the 50 percent tax bracket but $35,834 if the money was placed in a tax-sheltered program.

The list of possible retirement plans available through financial institutions such as banks, savings and loan associations, credit unions, mutual funds, brokerage firms, and insurance companies reads like a can of alphabet soup: IRA, TDA, SPDA, and HRIO. In addition, the federal government provides FICA. This section will review the major retirement plans available and suggest some key questions you should consider.

### Social Security (FICA)

For almost all salaried and many self-employed individuals social security tax is mandatory under the Federal Insurance Contributions Act. Both employee and employer contribute an equal amount, based on the employee's income and a fixed tax rate. Both figures keep increasing: for example in 1977 both employee and employer paid the government 5.85 percent of the employee's first $16,500 and by 1987 the figures are expected to be 7.15 percent of the employee's first $42,600. The self-employed clinician who is incorporated is required to pay the entire contribution toward his or her social security and the solo practitioner too has to pay the total FICA, though at a somewhat lower tax rate, (for example, the individual rate in 1978 was 8.19 percent, while the combined employee-employer rate was 12.10 percent. The difference is about 4 percent.)

Although there is considerable controversy surrounding the social security retirement plan, most Americans are covered by it and at present can expect to receive some retirement benefits when they reach age 62 or 65, whichever they elect. Most financial planners consider social security benefits the first step of a retirement plan and suggest other retirement plans to supplement social security income.

### Keogh Retirement Plans (HR–IO)

The Self Employed Individual's Tax Retirement Act of 1962 provided self-employed individuals the opportunity to build a financially secure retirement while realizing valuable tax advantages. The following summarizes highlights of the Act:

- Three classes of employees are defined:
  (1) Owner-employees—self-employed individuals owning a trade or business and partners whose capital interest is in excess of 10 percent.
  (2) Other self-employed—persons who are members of a partnership but whose interest in the partnership is 10 percent or less.
  (3) Regular employees
- Owner-employees may contribute up to 15 percent of earned income or $15,000, whichever is less.

- The plan must also cover other full-time employees, with contributions for them vested immediately. Contributions of at least the same percentage made for owner-employees must be made for all other eligible employees.
- Contributions to the plan are deductible as a business expense.
- Must have a specific Plan and a Plan Trustee.
- Participants incur no tax on contributions or earnings of the plan until benefits are received.
- Participants can use life insurance and annuity contracts, as well as invest in banks, savings and loans, mutual funds, government bonds.

One major disadvantage often cited of Keogh plans is the requirement that employers covered by the plan must provide employees with a similar plan by contributing the same percentage of the employers' plan for them.

Moneys placed in a Keogh plan are available upon retirement at age 55. If money is withdrawn at an earlier time, substantial financial penalties are imposed by the Internal Revenue Bureau. Currently, a self-employed clinician can set aside a maximum $25,000 annually.

**Individual Retirement Accounts (IRAs)**

IRAs have been a traditional retirement avenue of employed individuals who do not have retirement programs available or those self-employed individuals who choose not to invest in a Keogh plan. Current tax laws permit self-employed individuals to have both Keogh and IRA plans, but remember that the investment ceiling of an IRA is considerably lower than a Keogh plan. Furthermore, with the pressures of inflation, it may take $1 million or more for you to live as comfortably in retirement as during your working years. If inflation averages 10 percent a year, in 35 years $1 million would equal approximately $35,000 in today's dollars. At an 8 percent average inflation rate, $1 million would be worth $68,000 in the year 2017 in terms of today's purchasing power.

It is also important to consider that if inflation falls off well below 10 percent, it is unlikely that high interest rates will prevail long enough for an IRA to "make you a millionaire."

Assuming a return of two or three percentage points above the inflation rate is a more conservative way of looking at the return of IRA investments. For example, an inflation-adjusted return of 2 percent on an annual $2,000 investment would grow to approximately $100,000 at the end of 35 years, at 3 percent to $121,000.

Business institutions have been aggressively pursuing IRA moneys with enticing advertisements promising a two-income family that by contributing

$4,000 annually for 30 years to an IRA that earns 12 percent compound interest, they can retire as millionaires. However, IRAs are not for everyone, even though everyone may contribute. For example, if you anticipate being in a very high tax bracket after retirement (i.e., 50 percent), then tax-free bonds may be a better consideration.

It is also permissible to transfer the assets of one IRA plan from one trustee to another, or roll over your funds from a retirement fund into an IRA account. The Internal Revenue Service allows such transfers without a tax penalty. If you receive a lump sum payment from a retirement plan, you have up to 60 days to roll over funds into an IRA without being liable for taxation. Note that, although federal regulations permit transfer of an IRA to gain maximum interest rates, the financial institution may not.

The following are some highlights of IRA pension programs:

- An individual may establish an IRA and make a contribution to it during a taxable year unless covered under a qualified retirement plan during the year.
- An employer can set up an IRA for employees under certain conditions.
- An individual may contribute during a taxable year up to
  (1) an amount equal to 15 percent of compensation includible in gross income for the taxable year, or
  (2) $2,000, whichever is the lesser amount.
- An individual will be deemed to have made a contribution on the last day of the preceding taxable year if it is made not later than 45 days after the end of such taxable year.
- Special tax-favored treatment is provided for roll-over amounts from other qualified retirement plans.
- An individual's interest in IRA must be nonforfeitable.
- Participants incur no tax on contributions or earnings of the plan until benefits are received.
- Participants can use annuities, retirement income, and certain endowment contracts that meet established requirements.
- Distributions prior to age 59½ are subject to penalty. The IRA must be distributed not later than the close of the taxable year in which age 70½ is attained.
- A custodian or trustee is needed unless the contract is issued by an insurance company. The contract does not need to be submitted to IRS but Form 5329 must be filed each year.

- At the time of delivery the seller of an IRA must furnish the purchaser, in a written disclosure statement, information that is required by IRS regulations.
- The Tax Reform Act of 1976 made provision for an IRA for a spouse of an individual who establishes an IRA provided the spouse has no compensation and is not covered as a member of a qualified retirement plan. A spouse IRA requires certain changes in some of the provisions that are included in an IRA set up for only one individual.

**Corporate Pension Plans**

While clinicians who incorporate are not eligible for a Keogh pension plan, they can provide tax-sheltered retirement plans through their corporation. Indeed, as previously discussed in Chapter 2, this is one of the primary reasons for incorporating. Stock bonus, pension, or profit-sharing plans are available as corporate retirement plans. Furthermore, there are no maximum contributions an employer can make and moneys contributed to retirement plans are looked upon as a corporate expense by the Internal Revenue Service. These plans have much flexibility, complexity, and cover all members of the corporation. Thus careful consideration and legal and accounting consultation are required prior to establishing such arrangements.

**Tax-Deferred Annuities (TDAs)**

Sheltering income through tax-deferred annuities is popular with clinicians who spend part of their time consulting to or being salaried by public schools, religious, charitable, or nonprofit organizations such as community mental health centers or child guidance clinics. Tax-deferred annuities were designed to stimulate retirement savings and to offer significant tax advantages for eligible individuals.

Contributions, subject to IRS limits, are set aside and invested to build a fund to provide retirement benefits. Amounts contributed through your employer are currently deductible from income subject to federal tax, and these contributions, along with the interest earned, are not taxed until distributed, typically at retirement. At that time you will probably be in a lower tax bracket, which means you could realize an additional tax savings.

There are two basic methods by which you can contribute to a TDA. The first is by taking a reduction in salary. Under this method you must enter into a salary reduction agreement with your employer and have your employer forward the amount of the reduction, up to 16-2/3 percent of your salary, to the organization through which the TDA is established. The second method is by foregoing an increase in salary. With this method you can request that in lieu of a salary increase your employer contribute an amount of up to 20 percent of your salary to the TDA.

There are also higher makeup contribution formulas that can be used by individuals who have not taken advantage of a TDA during prior years of eligibility, as well as special contribution rules that can be exercised by employees of educational institutions, hospitals, and home health service agencies.

No matter which method you elect it is important to remember that only contributions forwarded directly by your employer are excludable for federal income tax purposes. Contributions you make directly to the TDA are not eligible for this exclusion. Interest earned on all contributions is not taxed until such time as you withdraw your funds or begin to receive income in the form of a monthly annuity.

If you change employers and are still eligible for the TDA, with your new employer's permission, you may continue having contributions placed into your existing TDA contract. You must, however, sign a new salary reduction agreement with your employer. You can also continue making contributions if you terminate your employment and are no longer eligible for the TDA. These contributions, however, are not eligible for the federal income tax exclusions, although the interest earned will continue to accumulate tax deferred.

Your funds can be withdrawn at any time but normally you will not want to do so until retirement. At that time you may elect to receive the entire value of your TDA in one lump sum or in the form of a monthly annuity income. The payments you receive, minus any contributions you made directly, are taxable in full as ordinary income. However, if you elect monthly annuity payments, they are taxed only as you receive them. This way the tax liability is spread over the entire payout period.

## Single-Premium Deferred Annuity (SPDAs)

A relatively new and sophisticated approach to retirement investing has been provided by insurance companies in the form of a single-premium deferred annuity. The minimum single investment is usually $5,000. The interest is tax sheltered, and since the individual has already paid taxes on the original investment there are no special IRS restrictions as on IRA or Keogh plans. Furthermore, you are permitted to withdraw up to 10 percent of your SPDA annually without a tax liability.

A single-premium deferred annuity plan offered by such insurance companies as Penn Mutual provides guaranteed safety of principal investment, withdrawal privileges, and no sales charge. Although this retirement plan is highly flexible and very attractive, the minimum large initial investment can be a drawback to practitioners entering practice.

**Choosing the Right Plan**

When considering tax-sheltered retirement programs, whether IRA, Keogh, or TDA, you'll want to note the following factors:

- Type of investment institution—Institutions such as banks provide the most conservative and 100 percent insured investment; brokerage firms are among the riskiest.
- Interest rates—It is important to know whether the interest rates will be compounded, and if so, how: daily, quarterly. Furthermore, ask for how long the rates are in effect and are there minimum rates that are guaranteed, or a bail-out clause if the renewal rate falls below a guaranteed interest rate.
- Minimum initial investment—There is a wide spectrum of minimum deposits required ranging from none for some IRAs to $5,000 for single-premium deferred annuities. Some IRAs permit you to add to your account in minimum increments of $50 or $100; others require single payments for a certificate that runs for a particular length of time.
- Charges and fees—Some individual retirement accounts are front, rear, or front and rear loaded. Front loaded funds pay a commission at the beginning, reducing the amount invested; and rear loaded funds subtract a charge from the total amount prior to payout. Some retirement plans charge a penalty if the funds are withdrawn prematurely or before the account has been in effect a certain number of years. For example, Charter Security Life Insurance Co. (New York) charges a 7 percent fee if the money is withdrawn in the first year and scales down to zero after seven years.

  Group retirement plans usually carry neither a front nor a rear load charge; and if you remain in the plan for a minimum number of years, usually seven or ten, there is also no withdrawal fee. However, like all group plans, if you leave the group, or if its master group plan is terminated, you can no longer continue sheltering your money with the group. If you choose a company that has a number of plans, there may be a transfer fee. A transfer fee refers to the cost of shifting plans, for example, IRA resources from one fund to another within the same institution.

- Fixed and variable plans—Fixed interest plans are similar to whole life insurance in that the annuitant knows the amount his or her tax-sheltered plan will yield after a fixed period of years. Variable plans are unpredictable and depend on the value of the portfolio of the plan invested in at the time of retirement. It is similar to owning stock in a company.

When I discussed a number of "common business headaches" in Chapters 2 and 3, I suggested consulting with an accountant and a lawyer early in your practice. Managing money, investments, and retirement funds requires time and expertise. If you have neither time, expertise, nor interest in finance, then have a consultation with an independent financial advisor or arrange a meeting with a bank for a free discussion of the many ways you can build up a retirement nest egg while taking advantage of tax benefits. One final word of caution—there is no free lunch!

## GLOSSARY OF COMMON FINANCIAL TERMS

**ADB**—Accidental Death Benefit.

**Diversifier**—a retirement plan whereby a trustee can respond to a broad range of investment alternatives and make it easy for the plan sponsor to use them with confidence.

**Estate Plan**—proper use of estate assets to minimize estate taxes and estate shrinkage.

**Front Load**—commission is subtracted from the amount to be invested prior to investing.

**Funding Media**—the type of investment being done by a trustee on behalf of a retirement plan.

**Guaranteed Renewable**—referring to disability income where a policy is guaranteed to be renewed every year at the same rate, regardless of number of claims.

**HR-IO**—self-employed individual's retirement plan (Keogh).

**IRA**—Individual Retirement Account.

**Noncancelable**—cannot be canceled by carrier.

**PC**—professional corporation.

**Pension Plan**—fixed payment on behalf of plan members each year after retirement.

**Profit Sharing Plan**—same as pension plan, with the major exception being that amounts depend on profits.

**Rear Load**—Commission is subtracted from the total amount accumulated prior to payout.

**SPDA**—Single-premium deferred annuity.

**Split Funded Retirement Plan**—Pension money is divided into two segments: an investment portion and a life insurance portion.

**Tax-Deductible**—subtractable from currently taxed income.

**Tax-Deferred**—not currently taxed, as money generated by investments that is not distributed until retirement.

**Transfer Fee**—cost of shifting retirement funds from one plan to another within the same institution.

**Trustee**—one who administers a retirement plan for future retirees.

**TSA**—Tax Sheltered Annuities.

**Withdrawal Penalty**—cost that has to be paid if funds are withdrawn prematurely.

**WP**—Waiver of Premium. Premiums are waived in the event of total and permanent disability of client after four months of the contract being in effect.

## SUMMARY

Independent practitioners must provide their own fringe and retirement benefits. The following insurance and pension needs were detailed in this chapter:

- income
- health
- life
- professional liability
- retirement

# References


American Medical Association. *Principles of medical ethics.* Washington, D.C.: Author, 1957.

American Psychological Association. *Ethical standards for psychologists* (Rev. ed.). Washington, D.C.: Author, 1977.

American Psychological Association. *Specialty guidelines for the delivery of services by clinical psychologists.* Washington, D.C.: Author, 1980.

Beck, A.T., Rush, A.J., Shaw, B.F., & Emery, G. *Cognitive therapy of depression.* New York: Guilford Press, 1979.

Bergin, A.C., & Suinn, R.M. Individual psychotherapy and behavior therapy. In M.R. Rosenzweig & L.W. Porter (Eds.), *Annual Review of Psychology.* Palo Alto, Calif.: Annual Review, 1975.

Boneau C.A., & Cuca, J.M. An overview of psychology's human resources: Characteristics and salaries from the 1972 APA survey. *American Psychologist,* 1974, *29,* 821–840.

Brodsky, S.L., & Robey, A. On becoming an expert witness: Issues of orientation and effectiveness. *Professional Psychology,* 1972, 173–176.

Bromberg, W. *The uses of psychiatry and the law.* Westport, Conn.: Quorum Books, 1979.

Campbell, M., & Small, A.M. Chemotherapy. In B. Wolman, J. Egan, & A.O. Ross (Eds.), *Handbook of treatment of mental disorders in childhood and adolescence.* Englewood Cliffs, N.J.: Prentice-Hall, 1978.

Cass, L.K., & Thomas, C.B. *Childhood pathology and later adjustment.* New York: Wiley, 1979.

Cautela, J.R., & Wisocki, P.A. Thought stopping procedure. *The Psychological Record,* 1977 *27,* 255–264.

Choca, J. *Manual for clinical psychology practice.* New York: Brunner-Mazel, 1980.

Dorken, H., & Webb, J.T. 1976 third party reimbursement experience: An interstate comparison by insurance carriers. *American Psychologist,* 1980, *35,* 355–363.

Ellis, A. *The essence of rational psychotherapy: A comprehensive approach to treatment.* New York: Institute for Rational Living, 1970.

Eysenck, H.J. The effects of psychotherapy. *International Journal of Psychiatry,* 1965, *1,* 99–178.

Fassler, J. *Helping children cope.* New York: Free Press, 1978.

*Federal tax guide.* Chicago: Commerce Clearing House, 1983.

Ferber, A., Mendelsohn, M., & Napier, A. (Eds.). *The book of family therapy.* New York: Science House, 1972.

Freud, S. Further recommendations in the techniques of psycho-analysis. *Collected Papers* (Vol. II). London: Hogarth Press, 1953.

Gottfredson, G.D., & Dyer, S.E. Health service providers in psychology. *American Psychologist,* 1978, *33,* 314–339.

Graziano, A.M. (Ed.). *Behavior therapy with children.* Chicago: Aldine/Atherton, 1971.

Graziano, A.M. Behavior therapy, In B. Wollman, J. Egan, & A.O. Ross (Eds.), *Handbook of mental disorders in childhood and adolescence.* Englewood Cliffs, N.J.: Prentice-Hall, 1978.

Guggenheim, P.D. The juvenile offender. *Bulletin, Area 11, American Psychiatric Association,* March 1979.

Haakenson, R. *You are the next speaker.* Philadelphia: Smith, Klein, & French Laboratories, 1962.

Halpern, W.I. The medication clinic in the spectrum of children's services. *Diseases of the Nervous System,* 1977, *38,* 667–690.

Halpern, W.I., & Kissel, S. *Human resources for troubled children.* New York: Wiley Interscience, 1976.

Harrower, M. *The practice of clinical psychology.* Springfield, Ill.: Charles C Thomas, 1961.

Hollister, L.E. *Clinical use of psychotherapeutic drugs.* Springfield, Ill.: Charles C Thomas, 1974.

Huffman, E.K. *Medical record management.* Berwyn, Ill.: Physicians Record Co., 1972.

Johnson, A.M. School phobia: Discussion. *American Journal of Orthopsychiatry,* 1957, *27,* 307–309.

Kissel, S. Mothers and therapist evaluate long term and short term child therapy. *Journal of Clinical Psychology,* 1974, *36,* 296–299.

Krasner, L. Behavior therapy. In P.H. Mussen & M.R. Rosenzweig (Eds.), *Annual Review of Psychology,* Palo Alto, Calif.: Annual Review, 1971.

Leventhal, T., & Weinberger, G. Evaluation of a large scale brief therapy program for children. *American Journal of Orthopsychiatry,* 1975, *45,* 119–134.

Levitt, E.E. Research in psychotherapy with children. In A. Bergin & S. Garfield (Eds.), *Handbook of psychotherapy and behavior changes.* New York: Wiley, 1971.

Lewin, M.H. *Establishing and maintaining a successful professional practice.* Rochester, N.Y.: Professional Development Institute, 1978.

Liebenson, H.A., & Wepman, J.M. *The psychologist as expert witness.* Wilmette, Ill.: Callaghan & Co., 1964.

MacDonald, J.M. Psychiatry and the criminal (2nd ed.). Springfield, Ill.: Charles C Thomas, 1969.

Mahoney, M.J. *Cognitive and behavior modification.* Cambridge, Mass.: Ballinger Publishing Co., 1974.

Meichenbaum, D.B. *Cognitive-behavior modification: an integrative approach.* New York: Plenum, 1977.

Mellsop, G.W. Psychiatric patients seen as children and adults: Childhood predictors of adult illness. *Journal of Psychology and Psychiatry,* 1972, *13,* 91–101.

Messer, S.B., & Winokur, M. Some limits to the integration of psychoanalytic and behavior therapy. *American Psychologist,* 1980, *35,* 818–827.

Miller, N. The scientist's responsibility for public information. *Society for Neuroscience,* 1978.

Minuchin, S., & Fishman, H.C. *Family therapy techniques.* Cambridge, Mass.: Harvard University Press, 1981.

NASW Register of Clinical Social Workers. *Code of ethics.* Washington, D.C.: National Association of Social Workers, 1978.

Natural Resource Center for Consumer and Legal Services. Dayton, Ohio: Bury Market Research, 1980.

Neher, J. (Ed.). *Current audiovisuals for mental health education.* Chicago: Marquis Academic Media, 1979.

O'Leary, K.D., & Wilson, G.T. *Behavior therapy: Application and outcome.* Englewood Cliffs, N.J.: Prentice-Hall, 1975.

Patterson, C.H. *Theories of counselling and psychotherapy* (3rd ed.). New York: Harper & Row, 1980.

Pressman, R.M. *Private practice—A handbook for the independent mental health practitioner.* New York: Gardner Press, 1979.

Psychotherapy finances. *Guide to psychotherapy.* South Orange, N.J.: Ridgewood Financial Institute, 1980.

Public Law 94–142. *Federal Register,* 1977.

Public Law 96–398. *Federal Register,* 1980.

Richman, J. Reporting diagnostic test results to patients and their families. *Journal of Projective Techniques and Personality Assessment,* 1967, *31,* 62–71.

Robins, C.N. Follow-up studies of behavior disorders in children. In H.C. Quay & J.S. Werry (Eds.), *Psychopathological disorders of children.* New York: Wiley, 1972.

Satir, V. *Co-joint family therapy.* Palo Alto, Calif.: Science and Behavior Books, 1967.

Shrybman, J., & Halpern, W.I. The mental health clinician's day in court. Workshop, Rochester Mental Health Center, March 1979.

Slovenko, R. *Psychiatry and law.* Boston: Little, Brown, 1973.

Stetler, C.J., & Moritz, A.R. *Doctor & patient and the law.* St. Louis: C.V. Mosby & Co., 1962.

Thorpe H.S., & Halpern, W.I. Pediatrics and a community child guidance clinic. *Pediatrics,* 1965, *36,* 773–781.

Watzlawick, P., Weakland, J., & Fisch, R. *Change: Principles of problem formation and problem resolution.* New York: Norton, 1974.

Wellner, A.M., & Mills, D.H. How many health service providers in psychology? (Register Research Report No. 1). Unpublished manuscript, Council for the National Register of Health Service Providers in Psychology, 1977.

Wells, R.A., Dilkes, T.C., & Triuelli, N. The results of family therapy: A critical review of the literature. *Family Process,* 1972, *11,* 189–207.

White, R.W. Ego and reality in psychoanalytic theory: A proposal regarding independent ego energies. *Psychological Issues.* 3, monograph 11, 1963.

Wolman, B.B., Egan, J., & Ross, A.O. (Eds.). *Handbook of treatment of mental disorders in childhood and adolescence.* Englewood Cliffs, N.J.: Prentice-Hall, 1978.

Yates, A.J. *Behavior therapy,* New York: Wiley, 1970.

# Index

## A



## B

## C



## D



## E

## F



## G



## H



## I



## J



## K

## V



## W



## Y

# About the Author

STANLEY KISSEL received his Ph.D. from the University of Buffalo in 1961. Dr. Kissel is the Chief Psychologist at the Children and Youth Division of the Rochester Mental Health Center, Incorporated, and maintains an independent practice. He is a Diplomate in Clinical Psychology, American Board of Professional Psychology, a Fellow of the American Orthopsychiatric Association, and a past President of the Genesee Valley Psychological Association. The author of numerous publications, his most recent books include *Human Resources for Troubled Children,* 1976 (with Werner Halpern); *A Teacher's Guide to Understanding the WISC-R,* 1978 (with Pearl Kissel); and *An Eclectic Approach to Family Therapy,* 1980.